Appetite for Life is an extremely valuable resource to people struggling with eating disorders. It helps them understand that they are not alone and that many others have experienced exactly what they are experiencing. It not only provides personal stories but information on how to access professional services if desired. The book also helps illustrate to the reader that treatment for an eating disorder will likely be long and complicated, but also instills hope by illustrating the steps necessary for successful treatment. Most professionals would also benefit from such stories, considering that eating disorders are some of the most complicated psychological disorders to understand and conceptualize.

—Donald E. Greydanus, MD
Professor, Pediatrics and Human Development
Michigan State University College of Human Medicine

Through the voices of six women and one man who won the battle with their eating disorder, *Appetite for Life* offers hope and courage to those who still struggle. The book also superbly describes the recovery process and provides guidance and practical advice for family members as well. I will recommend Margie Ryerson's book to all of my patients.

—Eleni Lantzouni, MD, FAAP
Pediatrician and Adolescent Medicine Physician with special interest in
Eating Disorders

Appetite for Life will touch the hearts of those suffering from an eating disorder. *Appetite for Life* goes to the best source possible—real people who have suffered from eating disorders—to help others understand, cope and win their own battle.

—Tom McMahon, Professor of Psychology
Author of *Teen Tips* and nationally syndicated parenting columnist

This book is a rare resource that brings a positive perspective from the patients' point of view to the task of telling stories to illuminate the journey through these illnesses. One of the great motivators for change is seeing someone else be successful with their problem. This book is a great resource for adolescents and adults who are looking for solace from others who have suffered and found their way towards healing. It will also serve a great need that parents have to understand these illnesses.

—Cheryl Appel, MD, FAAP

Appetite for Life

Appetite for Life

✦

Inspiring Stories of Recovery from Anorexia, Bulimia, and Compulsive Overeating

Margie Ryerson, MS, MFT

iUniverse, Inc.
New York Lincoln Shanghai

Appetite for Life
Inspiring Stories of Recovery from Anorexia, Bulimia, and Compulsive Overeating

iUniverse books may be ordered through booksellers or by contacting:

iUniverse
2021 Pine Lake Road, Suite 100
Lincoln, NE 68512
www.iuniverse.com
1-800-Authors (1-800-288-4677)

ISBN-13: 978-0-595-34755-1 (pbk)
ISBN-13: 978-0-595-79497-3 (ebk)
ISBN-10: 0-595-34755-X (pbk)
ISBN-10: 0-595-79497-1 (ebk)

Printed in the United States of America

For Vic, Laurel, Jen, Mom, and Stan

And in memory of my fathers, Victor A. Strasburger
and Arthur C. Strasburger

Contents

ACKNOWLEDGMENTS

My appreciation and thanks to: the seven inspirational people who volunteered their stories to help others; Alison Picard, literary agent, who provided so much help along the way; Liz Voisin, who transcribed the interviews with skill and enthusiasm; and Deb Waterhouse, MPH, RD, who graciously lent her time and expertise.

And special appreciation for their continuous support and encouragement to Vic, Laurel, and Jen; Marjorie C. Strasburger; Susan Strasburger; Victor C. Strasburger, MD; Stanley Goldberg; Roy Turpin; Jason Kalan; Andrea Pfeiffer; Linda Shafer; Myra Kramer; Fran Sparrow; Debbie Parelskin; Martha Fischer; Hillary Hoppock; Ann Elliott; Leslie Hamerling; Dorothy Stewart; Gail Levie; and to all my other friends, family, and colleagues.

INTRODUCTION

The Battle Within

It's hard to say good-bye, you know
To something you've depended on.
A comfort, a friend, and yet a foe
My eating disorder.

Each morning I awake these days
So glad to feel better
Yet nagging in my mind and heart
Those little voices chatter.

"You're fat, you're ugly, such a slob!
Those pounds have got to go."
I want to stumble back again
But forward I must go.

For letting my disorder win
Means never living fully.
It means just giving up on me
And that would be so silly.

So I just struggle on each day
Fighting, oh so mightily.
And I have faith I'll someday put
My eating disorder behind me.

(by a patient in a hospital eating-disorders program)

This poem reflects one young woman's struggle, will, and potential for change. Anyone who has suffered from an eating disorder understands just how difficult change can be. One of my patients described it as trying to jump off a very high diving board into a swimming pool the size of a picnic table; that's how scary it seemed to her. The first step is making the *decision* to change. Some people take a very long time before they can even get to this first jumping-off point. In my experience as a therapist, I have observed several reasons why individuals may finally decide to take the leap away from unhealthy, self-defeating thinking and behavior:

- *Hitting bottom.* Unfortunately, this scenario is a common one. Only by repeatedly experiencing a great deal of pain and suffering are some people able to decide there has to be a better way to live. These individuals are not masochists; they are simply holding on to what they know, what feels comfortable even in a negative way, because that is a natural tendency. There is a biological concept called *homeostasis* that explains this behavior. It describes the inclination of organisms to seek to maintain the status quo despite changes in environmental conditions. Some patients come in for therapy quite beaten down—after a painful divorce, serial job losses, worrisome medical symptoms, or alienation from family and friends.

- *Significant events.* Some women decide to work on their eating disorders when they want to become pregnant. Some have small children and want to be better parents and role models. One woman in her forties, with a sixteen-year history of bulimia, came to see me for help because she was invited to join some close friends on a six-month sailing trip the following year. She knew she would have little privacy if she went, but a trip such as this was a lifelong dream of hers. This opportunity provided her with the impetus to change. One young woman in this book made the decision to recover when she left home for college. She was able to break away from her former label of "anorexic" and develop a new identity.

- *Entering nurturing relationships.* Another woman in this book describes feeling that while she was growing up, no one in her family actually "saw" her or "knew" her. When she grew older and developed intimate, loving relationships with friends and with her husband, she was able to shed her compulsion to overeat. Having the support and security of loved ones enables some people to tackle the scary and difficult process of change.

- *Hearing others' stories through books, articles, or television, or by attending support groups.* My wish is that reading the personal, heartfelt stories in this book will provide you with hope, ideas, and inspiration to help you in your path to recovery.

Years ago I worked as a therapist in a hospital eating disorders treatment program that served as a vital resource for patients and their families. We ran separate groups for patients and families, and conducted individual and family therapy. In both my hospital work and my therapy practice, I have witnessed the enormous suffering eating disorders wreak on individuals and their families. I generally refer to both patients and therapists in this book as being female, for purposes of simplification, but there are increasing numbers of males being treated for eating disorders.

My work with "Molly," a 16-year-old with anorexia, prompted me to write this book. Molly came to see me in my therapy practice. As she grew stronger, she asked me for some reading suggestions so that she could read about others who had gone through problems similar to hers. Molly felt very isolated because of her eating disorder and did not wish to discuss it with anyone but me. Yet she needed the reassurance that she was really not alone in what she thought and felt, and that others who had been in the same situation had ultimately recovered. Happily, Molly has since recovered from anorexia. Since that time several years ago, when she requested a book like this, many more patients have expressed a similar desire to read of others' struggles and recoveries.

An eating disorder is a very personal, potentially embarrassing problem. Revealing it to others can feel like proclaiming to the world, "I think I'm fat, unattractive, and not good enough, and I'm afraid I can't control myself around food. I may stuff myself or deny myself, but my thoughts are mostly centered on what I eat, what I look like, what I weigh, and how my appearance compares to that of others."

Needless to say, in a society like ours, where image is highly important, not many people want to risk appearing "not okay." And much of the eating disorder behavior itself is a source of embarrassment: bingeing on huge quantities of food, usually very rapidly and messily; self-inducing vomiting; ingesting large amounts of laxatives or diuretics, resulting in an unsettled stomach and loose stools; hiding food; stealing food; and lying about food consumption.

It was surprisingly easy to find people who were willing to be interviewed for this book. Each person expressed a strong desire to help others by sharing his or her path to recovery. Many said they were further strengthened every time they repeated their story. I have changed names and other means of identification to protect their privacy.

As you read through these stories, you will notice how each individual found a variety of tools to aid in his or her recovery. No two people find identical means to help themselves become healthy. This concept is a hopeful one; if one approach isn't effective, there are many other possible solutions.

However, there are some unifying themes that run throughout these stories. First, each person came to the realization that he or she had a serious problem. Second, each made a decision to try to become healthy. Third, in the course of becoming healthy, each one experienced the up-and-down nature of recovery. Progress does not occur in a steady upward progression, but rather comes in fits and starts, in ups and downs. Tolerating these fluctuations is difficult and discouraging at times, but these individuals kept picking themselves up, dusting themselves off, and trying some more.

Finally, each person came to depend on others for support and assistance. Most turned to therapy, eating disorder programs, or community support programs, as well as to help from family and friends. An individual with an eating disorder usually has a very narrow perspective in the sensitive areas of self-image, food, weight, and body image issues, and interactions with others. Most would prefer to be able to recover completely on their own and not have to share their shame and private feelings with others. However, outside support and intervention are almost always essential to recovery.

You may be reading this book because either you or a loved one has an eating disorder. If so, here is what I hope you will gain from these pages:

- An understanding of some of the underlying conflicts associated with eating disorders.

- Compassion for yourself or loved one. Many individuals and their families blame themselves for this problem and, as a result, carry around a great deal of guilt and self-imposed anger. Unless you made a *conscious* decision to develop and suffer the effects of an eating disorder or you *intentionally* wanted your loved one to go through misery with an eating disorder, blame is irrelevant. I hope you can acknowledge that although we all could be better people in lots of ways, we are only human—which is to say, imperfect.

- The knowledge that blame is destructive, depressing, and self-defeating.

- A realization that you are not alone in your experiences.

- Ideas for treatment and recovery.

- A hopeful vision for your recovery. Individuals who succeed in combating this disorder typically become emotionally stronger; more energetic, creative, and insightful; and more compassionate toward themselves and others.

1

AN OVERVIEW OF EATING DISORDERS AND THEIR TREATMENT

Anorexia

Anorexia nervosa is a complex and potentially life-threatening disorder. It is characterized by a loss of 25 percent or more of body weight with no organic cause, a morbid fear of fatness, a distorted body image, and cessation of or failure to begin menstrual periods.

The term *anorexia* comes from the Greek word meaning "without appetite." Anorexics shun food, withdraw socially, deny they have problems, and continue to feel fat despite being thin from near starvation. They tend to be perfectionists, expecting and demanding only the best from themselves. Often there is ritualistic and compulsive behavior, such as overexercising, and a need for extreme orderliness and cleanliness.

Physical symptoms may include weakened vital signs, such as lowered blood pressure and pulse rate; cold extremities; electrolyte (chemicals which surround cell membranes) imbalance; thinning scalp hair; increased facial and body hair (lanugo), which grows in order to help conserve body heat; dry, flaky skin; constipation; insomnia; hyperactivity; and joint pain.

Over 90 percent of anorexics are women, usually between the ages of 12 and 30, but some develop it at an earlier or later age. The average incidence for teenage girls is approximately 1 in 100. Recovery time from this disorder can range from six months to many years. Sadly, some victims of anorexia die: the estimated mortality rate is between 3 to 5 percent. Causes of death are usually electrolyte imbalance (the cause of singer Karen Carpenter's death at age 32 from heart failure), malnutrition, infection (due to a weakened immune system), and suicide. Some anorexics struggle with various symptoms throughout their lives, but many are able to make a complete recovery.

Recently, a number of controversial Web sites have promoted anorexia as a lifestyle choice. Some sites encourage the eating disorder by offering tips on how to survive on two hundred calories a day, or how to hide weight loss from parents and doctors. Other sites feature doctored photo images of thin actresses and models, making them appear even skinnier. These photos, and others of real-life anorexics, are touted as examples of the ideal feminine physique. One theory behind the origination of these Web sites is that some anorexics create them as a means of escape and denial. The creators may suffer from such malnutrition that their perceptions are distorted. They truly believe that the starved, skeletal look of anorexia is attractive and desirable.

Bulimia

While anorexia receives more media attention, possibly because its effects are more visible and dramatic, bulimia is much more prevalent. It is estimated that there are 10 to 12 women (and, increasingly, men) with bulimia for every 1 with anorexia. Because most bulimics practice their eating disorder in secrecy while remaining close to a normal weight, it is difficult to determine the exact incidence.

Bulimia, a word derived from the Greek term meaning "ox hunger," is a compulsive cycle of starving, binge eating, and vomiting. Bulimics often look normal but exhaust their bodies, bingeing on as much as thousands of calories of food at one time, several times a day, then using laxatives or vomiting to purge. There are degrees of severity, as with any disorder. I have treated patients who were bulimic only once a month to those who had episodes between 12 and 15 times per day.

Medical consequences may include irregular heartbeat and electrolyte imbalance, a ruptured esophagus or stomach, erosion of tooth enamel, gum problems, severe dehydration, and irreversible kidney damage that can lead to death. Since bulimic behavior is sometimes coupled with other forms of substance abuse, such as heavy alcohol and drug use, it is difficult to determine an exact rate of mortality. Untreated depression and careless, accident-prone behavior also contribute to the mortality rate for bulimics.

Compulsive Overeating

Compulsive overeating, or binge eating without purging, in some cases has a pattern similar to bulimia. Some compulsive eaters alternate between restricting and bingeing, some overexercise, and some take laxatives or diuretics. Many, however, become overweight or even obese due to the large amount of calories ingested and the lack of counteractive behavior. Often the foods of choice are high in calories and fat content; sweets, bread, ice cream, and chips are the most popular. Compulsive overeating is more prevalent in our society than anorexia and bulimia, and the health consequences can be just as damaging: heart disease, diabetes, gall bladder problems, joint pain, depression, and a weakened immune system from poor nutrition.

CAUSES OF EATING DISORDERS

Unfortunately, there are no simple explanations for the onset of an eating disorder. The complexity and multiplicity of causes is usually a huge frustration to patients and families who are trying to get a grasp on this problem. Unlike medical conditions such as tuberculosis or hepatitis, which have known origins and predictable recovery patterns, eating disorders usually stem from a varying combination of biological, sociological, and psychological factors. Each patient's unique temperament, thought-process, genetic inheritance, and experiences play a role in the development of an eating disorder. We do know that many patients suffering from anorexia, bulimia, or compulsive overeating also suffer from clinical depression.

Quest for Thinness

It is known that many eating disorders originate with a diet. Since quick-loss, restrictive diets do not work, frustration and increased self-dissatisfaction can set in. Furthermore, frequent dieting attempts upset metabolic efficiency so that it becomes increasingly difficult to lose weight. After a strict regimen of deprivation, gaining back weight and often even more can lead some people to resort to extreme measures such as purging or laxative use. Attempts to restrict food intake often produce binge eating instead.

Anorexics, on the other hand, usually become too successful in their attempts to diet. They find they enjoy the feelings of control and mastery over their bodies, as well as the attention from others. In the beginning, the attention is usually positive and complimentary as they become thinner; later they revel in the attention and concern they receive for being too thin. But, ironically and improbably, as the disease becomes more insidious, anorexics resent expressions of concern about their physical appearance and health (after all, they want complete control over this area), but still crave attention and praise from others. As people withdraw from them because of fear, uncertainty, anger, or other uncomfortable feelings, anorexics become extremely isolated and even more entrenched in their disease process.

Why do so many people attempt to diet in the first place? There are many lengthy explanations to this question, but, briefly, here are a few significant factors. Over the past three or more decades our society has transmitted the message, largely through the media, that thin is beautiful. Not only that, but thinner is even more beautiful. As the saying goes, "You can never be too rich or too thin." Playmate centerfolds, fashion models, and Miss Americas are between 10 and 20 percent lower weight than the recommended norm for women their age and height. In magazine ads and television commercials, being thin is often associated with success, happiness, popularity, glamour, sexual desirability, and a host of other positive attributes. Unfortunately, it is the exception rather than the rule to find a woman of any age who is satisfied with her weight and size and shape of her body.

Women's attitudes toward their bodies have been strongly shaped by societal messages. Some of the qualities they ascribe to themselves when they are thin include enhanced strength, self-discipline, confidence, control, superiority to others, attractiveness, and ability to be outgoing. And women who are generally predisposed toward being larger or heavier than their thin ideal must struggle even harder to try to achieve their goals.

Some additional reasons women strive for thinness stem from hurtful or painful experiences. One former patient, a 27-year-old woman with a 12-year history of bulimia, spent many therapy sessions crying and raging against her recently deceased father for his negativity when she was younger. "Julia" was a chubby child whose father teased and belittled her because of her physique. He made it plain to her that he considered excess fat an indication of over-indulgence and lack of self-discipline. He put Julia on diet and exercise regimens from the time she was ten years old. By age fifteen, after many failed attempts to keep off an extra 20 pounds, Julia discovered purging and soon was caught up in the agonizing cycle of an eating disorder.

Another patient, "Megan," grew up feeling mediocre compared to her high-achieving older siblings. When she was seventeen, her parents divorced, and her boyfriend broke up with her. As Megan's world shattered around her, she took refuge in the only thing within her control—her body. Being the thinnest person in her family and at school gave her the sense of accomplishment she craved, and her preoccupation with losing weight allowed her to avoid dealing with painful events in her life.

An estimated 15 to 20 percent of eating disorder patients have been victims of sexual abuse. Some become anorexic as a way of shutting off their sexual identity, sexual feelings, and other strong feelings as well.

They look and feel asexual, a safe refuge from potential or actual outside threats.

Other Causes

Most eating disorders spring from a combination of factors. Personal traits, family dynamics, social functioning, and life-altering events all play significant roles in the evolution of anorexia, bulimia, and compulsive overeating. Frequently there is underlying moderate-to-severe depression.

Here are some of the most common determinants:

- A history of physical abuse, emotional abuse, or unstable family environment

- A personal or family history of substance abuse and/or depression

- Excessively controlling and intrusive parents

- Distant, aloof, or neglectful parents

- Poor self-image and social skills

- Teasing or ostracism as a child about weight or appearance

- Poor family communication—little sharing of feelings, especially anger and hurt

- Poor coping skills for problem solving

- Lack of firm, yet reasonable, limits and rules within the family

- Family overemphasis on appearance and achievement

- Poor assertiveness skills

- Lack of healthy emotional boundaries with a parent or sibling. This can lead to "enmeshment," an unhealthy relationship in which one individual's feelings, needs, and identity become entangled with those of another.

- Undeveloped identity, putting the individual at risk for overvaluing how others think and behave

- Unrealistically high expectations of self and others

- Creation of a false self—failure to behave in accordance with true thoughts and feelings. An example of this characteristic is the "superwoman syndrome" in which the individual denies having any problems, projecting an image of competence and well-being at all times.

TREATMENT AND RECOVERY

The standard treatment for eating disorders uses a combination of individual and family psychotherapy, nutritional counseling, and medical supervision. When there is underlying depression, antidepressant medication is prescribed. For some patients, group therapy can be helpful. The length of treatment varies, depending on the severity of the problem, the patient's degree of motivation to recover, family cooperation, and consistency in keeping appointments. One crucial component is that the patient likes and trusts the members of the treatment team, especially the individual therapist. The length of time for recovery from a well-entrenched eating disorder usually ranges from one to five years.

Hospitalization is necessary if a patient falls below 20 to 25 percent of her ideal body weight. Hospital programs differ, but most use behavioral techniques. The patient is placed on a high-calorie diet and is closely monitored during and after meals to eliminate opportunities for "food shrinkage." If a patient refuses to cooperate with this plan, she receives a gastronasal feeding tube through which liquid nourishment is inserted with a direct route to the stomach. Such resistant patients have enforced bed rest until they have gained enough weight to be able to exercise in safe increments. Some hospital programs offer therapy and nutritional counseling, but most are limited in scope by the length of time a patient can afford to stay. Hospitalization provides medical stabilization so that a patient can be healthy enough to benefit from outpatient treatment.

A recently adopted treatment for eating disorders is called the Maudsley method, named after the hospital in London that developed it. It is increasingly used as an alternative to hospitalization or residential treatment programs. This method focuses first on the eating problem and places parents in charge of overseeing the feeding of their child. Food is considered the medicine that parents need to administer. When the child is better nourished, she is then able to assume more control of her own feeding process. Eventually, individual and family therapy help address family, psychological, and developmental issues. The Maudsley method shows impressive results, and researchers are continuing to evaluate its efficacy. However, there are certain drawbacks to this approach: it is less effective with older adolescents, adults, and bulimics, and in families with enmeshed parent-child relationships.

Another form of treatment is a residential program. This is an alternative for those who are well enough not to require hospitalization, but who still need more care than several medical and counseling appointments a week can provide. Residential treatment programs offer a highly structured living situation. Patients reside in group homes, cottages, or dormitories with live-in supervisors. Staff members also include psychologists, physicians, and teachers. Residents follow a daily schedule with activities such as individual therapy, group therapy, expressive therapy (art, music, dance), nutritional counseling, meditation, journal writing, exercise, yoga, and living skills (shopping, cooking, budgeting, personal grooming, etc.). Programs usually require families to participate in family education and therapy as well.

As you will see in the following stories, some people recover with the help of programs such as Overeaters Anonymous, religious or spiritual beliefs and affiliations, and consistent support from family and peers. Most people make significant progress with ongoing psychotherapy and nutritional counseling, but not everyone chooses or benefits from these forms of treatment. There is not one "right" way to recover from an eating disorder; it is a personal path, much like the one taken by each of the seven people in these pages.

2

AMY

Amy is a 24-year-old high school teacher who struggled with her eating disorder for six years. She had anorexia with bouts of bingeing. Amy has been symptom-free for more than two years.

My earliest memory of feeling too fat was the summer before third grade. My family and I were visiting friends in Wisconsin. I was really skinny then, but for some reason I just decided I wasn't going to eat anymore. My mother forced me to wear shorts and I was really upset about that. I remember thinking, "I'm not going to wear them, you can't make me. I'm too fat, I'm too disgusting." I would hit my thighs to see them jiggle and say, "Look it, I'm fat." I had bruises on my thighs from trying to prove they were fat. I remember going to a baseball game and spending the entire time in the bleachers trying to sit up straight so that my legs wouldn't touch each other. I went that whole day feeling horrible when I shouldn't have. The feeling of being too fat lasted that whole summer, but when I returned to school in the fall I felt back to normal. To this day, my mother makes fun of how I was then.

I never got along well with my mother. She told me that from conception we didn't click, that we didn't like each other for nine months. She was nauseous throughout the pregnancy and pretty miserable. Then, when I was born she thought I didn't like her because I was crying and irritable and didn't like to be held. She basically gave me to my father and said, "Here, you take care of her because I can't."

My father raised me emotionally. There was no love from my mother's side. She would do car pools and stuff, but my dad is where I got one hundred percent of the love. When my sister was born four years later, she and my mom bonded. My sister is very loving and giving and more emotional than I am. I don't like to be touched as much and am more independent. So my mom and sister bonded and my dad and I bonded, and my sister and I didn't get along at all, ever. I remember my parents' explanation for having a sister was that I was a spoiled brat and needed to learn how to share, and that the only way I was going to learn how to share was if I had to share with a sibling. But I didn't share at all willingly. I have my own space and nobody comes into it, compared to my sister who gave everything and still does.

I put a higher value on my sister's personality. I think she's a better person in the sense that she is so willing to give to other people. That was something I had to learn. It didn't come naturally. My mother couldn't handle that, the thought that I was so distant and so independent. So as I got older, my mother and I just got more and more evil toward each other, and I basically did not want to have anything to do with her. She was very wicked about everything. She would snap at me at any moment. Everything had to be perfectly clean, like don't touch this and don't leave a spot of anything anywhere. When I was younger she would suddenly get furious with me and slap me. I was always physically afraid of her because she's a really big woman, and she would just come into my room and attack me. I didn't fight back. I would just curl up and go into a corner. So when I got older, I tried very hard to have my own life and not speak to her and avoid contact with her as much as possible. She just hated me more for trying to avoid her.

My dad is a chemical engineer and my mom has always been a homemaker. We never had much contact with my dad's parents, and they both died by the time I was thirteen. My mother's father is a retired scientist and has suffered from bad episodes of depression throughout his life. He had many episodes when my mother was growing up. He considered emotions a bad thing and would explain them away as chemical reactions in your brain. You're only feeling this emotion because of a synapse connection, that kind of thing. I think he used this rationale in order to stay constant and not give in to his depression. But everyone around him had to stay that way too. He's been institutionalized several times recently for his depression. I don't know how my grandmother and mom got along while she was growing up, but they're best friends now. I don't like my maternal grandmother. She definitely sides with my mother and says that my mother has done everything right, and I am always wrong.

My mother has been on anti-depressants at some point, so it is definitely possible that she suffers from depression and low self-esteem. That's probably why she took it so personally that I didn't love her, and it affected her self-esteem that she wasn't strong enough to be okay with herself. Now I also realize that she was jealous of me and all that I had going for me in my life as I grew up. She was also jealous because my father loved me more than he loved her. My dad and I are a lot alike, and he and my mom are totally different. My only explanation for why they are still married is that divorce is not an option for him. He swore he would always have a perfect marriage and never get divorced, and he won't.

My father is incredibly passive. Mom is the domineering one, and he just tries to placate her. He wishes that we could all get along and be the perfect happy family. He and I have never had an argument, ever. He is very caring and understanding and I just love him. He's the middleman in the family. When he's talking to me he presents my mother's side, and I am sure that when he is talking to her, he presents my side. He tries to make us understand because we don't talk to each other. He would like for me to make amends and come back into the family unit.

Even though I was pretty miserable and unhappy while I was growing up, I don't remember feeling fat after the experience in third grade until high school. I'd always been involved in sports, especially swimming and soccer. Then in high school I started playing tennis, and by junior year I was the number one seed on our tennis team. I also got into modeling for a local department store, for their print ads. I was 5'6" and weighed about 120 pounds. I remember wanting to weigh 118 pounds and not more than 120, and getting on the scale every day. I wanted my body to look perfect.

When I look back, I realize that I was always incredibly restricted with food. In every sport I played really hard, and I felt like the only time I was allowed to eat was if I exercised. My justification for eating was that my body needed food because I exercised it off. I only ate small portions and never ate desserts. I didn't feel good about myself because I didn't have many friends, but I did feel good about the way I looked and about being so good at tennis. I was blonde, tan, and buff.

But I didn't know how to eat normally. I didn't know what a normal amount of food was because my family didn't eat in a healthy way. My dad always ate junk food and snacked a lot. His side is naturally really tall and slender, and that's how I am naturally. My mother was always overweight and dieting, and we didn't have regular meals. We would have cereal for breakfast, nobody ate lunch, and dinner was really small portions because Mom was dieting. I learned that food was not okay, that you are not supposed to eat, and if you did, you should feel guilty about it. I just internalized these feelings about food and never questioned why I felt this way. Food was inherently evil and you were supposed to avoid it at all costs.

I felt in control of my eating until senior year. I was making straight A's in school, was a tennis star, had a few boyfriends on and off, but the situation at home got worse. I tried to have as little contact with my mother as possible because she would accuse me of all kinds of bad things which were untrue: going to wild parties, doing drugs, etc. I would get up in the morning and leave for school an hour early, at 6 A.M., before my mother got out of bed. After school I'd practice tennis until sundown and then go eat at a boyfriend's house. When I came home I would just go straight to my room. On weekends I'd run five miles, do Jane Fonda aerobics exercise for one and a half to two hours, and play tennis the rest of the day.

Well, I wound up coming down with mononucleosis. I hadn't been feeling very energetic and for the first time had to push myself to exercise. One time I passed out doing Jane Fonda. My body couldn't handle it and I didn't want to go running, but I still made myself. I was in tennis tournaments and knew that I wasn't performing well enough, even though I was giving 110 percent. I kept thinking I was just being lazy and wacky.

I was diagnosed with mono and had to stay in bed at home. The first day of bed rest I remember thinking how I was so pissed because I had chocolate the night before and now I couldn't get rid of it. I was mad that I had eaten it. Now it was stuck in my body permanently. I really felt that I was freaking out. There was no way I was going to eat. I was stuck home alone with my mother all day. There was nothing to do but watch TV and eat. So I planned breakfast, lunch and dinner, and I'd have a piece of toast and cottage cheese and carrots and grapes in very small amounts. I'd spend an hour eating, extremely slowly, and four hours planning what I would eat.

My mom, of course, would try to get me to eat more. But I always thought it was a conspiracy to get me fat because she was fat at the time. I thought that if I had her dinner, she would put extra butter on there just to make me fat. What was really scary was that she used to be as thin as me in high school.

After awhile I became so weak and dehydrated that I had to be fed intravenously. At that point it was obvious I was anorexic. I refused to eat because I felt there were already too many calories going into me through the IV. There was no eating disorders program at the hospital. A nutritionist came to talk to me, to tell me I needed to eat, and I just said no. I weighed between 90 and 92 pounds at that point.

I saw my family doctor three times while I had mono, but he didn't clue in that I was anorexic. I also saw a thyroid doctor because my parents thought a thyroid disorder might be the cause of the weight loss.

No one diagnosed my condition as anorexia. I bought some books on eating disorders and told my Dad, "This is me, this is so me." He said, "No, you're fine." I said, "But I obsess about food all the time." And he still kept saying, "You're fine, don't worry. I know you think that you have an eating disorder, but you don't." He was trying to be supportive, but he just didn't believe me.

I missed almost the whole last semester of high school, staying at home with mono, and nothing much changed that summer before college. I picked a college about a thousand miles from home because I wanted to get far away. When I arrived at school I weighed about 92 pounds. I didn't really want to, but I went through sorority rush because people kept telling me that I was so nonsocial that I'd never meet anyone in that university if I didn't. But sororities are not my thing. So I went through, and one of the days each sorority had food in every room. They had candies and chocolates and chocolate-covered strawberries and amazing food. I love chocolate, so I gorged. I totally binged. And they loved me for it. They thought I was so cool because I was the only person who was eating. So I ate at every house and in every room. They told me, "You're so cool. You're so easy to get along with." And that started me bingeing for the whole year.

Suddenly I was eating lots of food and not exercising. I tried to run, but I was taking difficult classes and had to study hard, and there just wasn't time. I had stopped playing tennis because of the mono, and just never got back into it. So I felt disgusted with myself for two reasons—that I was eating and not exercising—and I got over 130 pounds freshman year. I had never been that heavy before.

I binged all day long. I wouldn't eat a huge amount at one time, but I couldn't go without having food in my mouth. I think it's what being addicted to drugs would be like—always searching for it, always knowing where it is, how you can get it, and planning when to eat it. The lowest point I ever had was that year because I just felt horrible and fat. By then I was about 5'8". I weigh more than 130 pounds now and I'm comfortable with myself, but then I felt just huge, like everybody was staring at me because I was so fat.

I couldn't control myself around food. There was a communal fridge in my dorm. If there was anything in there, it was mine. My roommate always had a bag with her leftover lunch, and I would always take it. She never confronted me on it, never said anything, but I ate it every single day. I didn't eat in front of other people. I couldn't tell anybody that I had this problem.

Despite this, my roommate and I were good friends, and I also had another good female friend. Until college, I had never had a close female friend. I never liked them, never trusted them, never got along with them. I hated my mother, so I hated all women. But in college I had much better friends than I ever had in high school, male and female.

That summer I stayed at school and met Mike. He was from an upper-class background and was very self-conscious about his looks and my looks. I had to look perfect all the time. It was interesting that he went out with me. He thought I was slender and okay enough, when I felt disgusting. What I hated was that he would have loved me in high school when I was so buffed and so athletic and so thin, but now I was just a blob. We had a sexual relationship after the first few weeks. I had only had sex twice before, with a boyfriend in high school, so I wasn't very experienced. I didn't enjoy sex with Mike because I was so ashamed of my body. I couldn't relax and enjoy myself. I was too self-conscious.

We made plans for me to go home with him for a visit at the end of the summer to meet his family and friends. He lived in a community by the beach, so I would have to be in a bathing suit. I don't know what caused it, but I stopped eating and lost 30 pounds within six weeks. It was still a nightmare, going home with Mike, because I felt so out of place. I didn't have the clothes. I didn't have the attitude. And I didn't have a body like all the incredibly athletic and incredibly thin women I met there.

I knew I had to get skinnier so I could finally be happy. Soon I was down to 90 pounds again, but I still felt I had to keep losing. I went to a family reunion and saw my dad. He said, "Oh, you've lost weight." And I said, "Yeah, aren't I sickly-looking? I really need help." He said something like, "Oh, you're just fine," and shrugged it off. I just went crying into the bathroom. I wanted his attention. I had done all this work for my dad and for Mike, and I figured the two men in my life I was closest to would know that I had a problem.

That's when I realized that if I was ever going to get completely over this, I would have to get really sick to get serious help. I started going to a medical clinic at school which had a really good eating disorder program. They had a nutritionist, a nurse, a doctor, and a therapist. I had to go get weighed and get my vitals taken three times a week. This was great. I loved the attention and felt so cool because I was so thin. That's exactly what I wanted. I was getting attention and my problem was getting acknowledged. They were obviously concerned about me and thought I was sick. I was so afraid I was going to be found out, that they would tell me, "Now you're really fine. You can go home." So I kept getting thinner so they would believe me. The doctor said that if I got below a certain weight I would have to go to the hospital. So I thought, "Yeah," and I did.

I was scared because I didn't know how being hospitalized would affect school. There was a part of me that was tentative, but it ended up being the best thing I could have done. I went into the eating disorders unit of a local hospital and stayed for two months. The first five weeks were inpatient, and the last three weeks I was an outpatient. Then I went to the hospital from 9 A.M. until after dinner.

When I first got there, I didn't want to be there at all. I was being a pill, a giant pill. I would pout and not participate, and I sat in a corner. I was very much a pain. I remember the first thing they made us eat was a muffin, and I spent an hour and a half trying to eat this muffin for breakfast the very first day. It's funny to look back on it now and think about how hard that was.

There were five other women in the program. I liked my roommate, Julia. At first, I didn't open up at all and thought to myself what bullshit all the psychotherapy was, just stupid stuff. But we had a dream analysis group, and I had a dream that was so revealing I had to share it. In the dream I was walking with Julia and other friends and going up a really steep hill. It was really beautiful, and then Julia turns around and says she's leaving. I say, "Don't go." She says, "Don't worry, I'll be back," and she didn't come back. So it was revealing in the sense that I've had a really hard life walking uphill—abandonment, people leaving. I told that in the group and began to open up.

I decided to try taking an antidepressant since they worked for the others in the program. I took Prozac and it worked great for me from day one, no side effects at all. I had been severely depressed for several years leading up to the hospitalization, and between therapy and the medication, I never had another period like that.

I dropped two classes and did my two other classes from the hospital. That was really hard because I was pretty much a straight A student. I worried about not doing well when I couldn't attend lectures and was busy all day doing therapy. By the end of the day I was so drained, and then I had to do hours of homework.

Once I stopped fighting it, the program gave me my recovery and it gave me self-esteem. Mostly, it taught me how to eat. I didn't know what a normal amount to eat was, or how to eat three meals a day. Most importantly it taught me how to eat, that I was supposed to eat, that I *deserved* to eat. I had to eat and it wasn't a negative thing.

In the beginning I was forced to eat the meals—types of food and quantities of food that no anorexic would ever put on her own plate. If I didn't eat, I would have to stay in bed and get tube-fed, and I know I didn't want that, especially after my awful experience with the IV when I had mono. I think it does have to be forced in the beginning because an anorexic would never get used to eating food otherwise. I spent hours eating some meals and stressing about it. We would all walk after every meal, and I would escape to go running every once in awhile. It was hard, but I did learn to get used to food being in my system and not feeling disgusting about it.

There was a 14-year-old girl named Meredith who was anorexic. It really helped that she was eating and telling me it was okay. Seeing another anorexic woman eat is so comforting. I felt like if she could do it, I could do it. And one of the therapists was a huge help. I didn't lift my eyes up when I was eating. I was so focused on the food. So, she said, "Okay, Amy, why don't you try having a conversation, why don't you look at me and we'll try to talk while you eat?" That was a totally foreign concept. I had to be taught how to do that.

Another thing that was difficult was that, even though I was really working the program hard, I was still obsessing about food. It was twenty-four hours a day, every second of the day where I was thinking about food. My therapist suggested that at the beginning of the day I allow myself a half hour to completely obsess, to get it all out, just max myself out on it. Then the rest of the day, whenever a thought came into my head I was supposed to say no, scream no.

Well, in the beginning I needed an hour in the morning. I remember being in the shower one morning and I was really focusing. I told myself to really obsess and think about the food and the fat, and just for a second my mind slipped to something else. I was like, stop, you're supposed to be focusing on the food. But I realized how hopeful that was. I had a thought that wasn't food, and that really hadn't happened for years. I really didn't think my mind could do that anymore. Then, whenever I had another second or two seconds I would write it down in my journal. Acknowledging it every time it happened increased the amount of time that it happened. I would think, "Wow, I went a whole five minutes today. Wow, that's a really long time."

Later, when I got out of the hospital, I wanted to know what other people thought about. Whenever I was with my friends I wanted to know what they were thinking about so I would know what I was supposed to be thinking about. It was such a good experiment because the boys were always thinking about sex. I would say, "Just tell me please…about sex?…okay, thanks." It was so funny. I did that for a long time, trying to figure out what to fill my head with if it's not food.

In the hospital we learned about the media's influence on us. We had lectures, went through magazine ads and articles, and learned to think critically. I was an economics major and very scientifically oriented, so at first I defended the advertisers. I thought the point was that they were just doing their job, trying to sell the product. But eventually I saw the negative things advertisers were doing. They use skinny, beautiful models so that the rest of us think, "I'm not perfect and I need to be perfect. I need to look like a model and I need to have all of these things." They exploit women's dissatisfaction with themselves to sell products. I don't buy fashion magazines anymore. I stay away from all that. I think my parents created an environment that was conducive to an addiction or to a disorder of some kind, but I think society defined what disorder I would have.

Another big thing I learned in the hospital was about all the family factors that led up to my anorexia. Their eating habits and attitudes, my mother's constant dieting, how that all played a role. It wasn't all my fault, I wasn't inherently, biologically just weird. I learned how I used my constant focus on food to avoid dealing with my problems. All my hurt and anger got poured into my relationship with my body and with food, instead of my relationship with my mother.

I have forgiven my mother for being a poor mother, but I don't want to be around her at all. She continues to put her own needs first and tries to manipulate me and others in our family to do what she wants. She doesn't respect any limits that I try to set. If she decides to visit me, she'll make arrangements whether I want her to or not. Sometimes she'll call my friends to try to find out what's going on in my life. When I had a therapist, she used to call her all the time to pump her for information. I just can't trust her. She has gossiped about me in malicious ways to other people and blames me for any problems in her own life. I feel that she's always looking for damaging evidence to use against me. She's always been so negative and critical of me, and I don't see any hope for change. It's too bad, but I'm better off without her in my life right now.

I definitely don't have any negative feelings toward my father and his role. You know, it's a bummer that he didn't stand up for me. I feel like if he would have kicked my mother out of the house, we would have all lived happily ever after, but that didn't happen. I feel so guilty about my dad. My dad is so unhappy, and I feel very much the cause of it all. He's still caught in the middle between my mother and me. But I have to protect myself and not allow my guilt over him to get in the way. It's clear to me now how I need to be, so that I won't ever get anorexic again.

After I left the hospital, I saw a private therapist once a week the rest of the time I was in college. I still had a lot of feelings to uncover and deal with, and I didn't feel completely recovered. I also joined a small weekly eating disorders support group and stayed with that for three years. The other three women and I got really close. It was a great feeling to have somewhere to go where people could easily understand what I was going through. Now, I don't feel like I need therapy, but I hope there will always be times in my life where I'm ready to really understand something more about myself.

Those first few years after the hospital were still a struggle. I noticed that whenever I felt down or bad about myself, I would automatically stop eating. That still seemed to be my natural response to problems. But after a day or two of restricting, I would remind myself that I never wanted to get sick again, so I would eat. I was so very much afraid of falling back into it. I mean horrified that I would get sick again and be miserable again. So that fear kept me fighting to stay in recovery.

I still felt too heavy much of the time, though, and not very attractive. I had learned not to get on a scale, so that helped, and I tried to concentrate on school, friends, and activities. I tried to stay in the comfort zone of not being too busy and stressed or too bored. Gradually, I took better care of myself and began to feel better, like I deserved to be happy and satisfied. And I didn't deserve being miserable.

Now that I've been healthy for over two years, I realize that *I* have to like and accept myself first so that I feel I deserve to be treated well by other people. For a few years in college, I was with different boyfriends who were nice to me in the beginning but then got really critical and judgmental. It's so wonderful feeling really positive about myself. When I talk to people now about what it was like to have an eating disorder, I really can't bring up the feelings. I eat well and I feel well, so it's hard to remember how miserable I was then.

This is my first year of teaching, and I like it so far. I'm still learning what I need to do, so sometimes it's overwhelming, but I really like the kids and the staff. I'm living with one roommate, a good friend from college. I don't have a boyfriend at the moment, but I'm happy anyway. That's really good for me. I used to *have* to be with someone or I couldn't be happy. I'm still on Prozac because when I went off it about a year ago, I started feeling slightly depressed and that scared me. But since there aren't any side effects, it really doesn't matter that much. I hope my story will help others feel that they can get over an eating disorder too. I've been asked to talk at a few schools and to other groups about my experience with anorexia, and I love doing that. I feel like I'm helping others and also myself at the same time.

3

LAURA

Laura is a 21-year-old college senior who suffered from anorexia, bulimia, and compulsive overeating for almost six years. She has been in recovery for two years.

I grew up in a suburb of a large city and lived in the same house all my life. My four sisters were twelve, thirteen, fifteen, and seventeen when I was born. When they all left the house it was like I was an only child, and when they came home it was like I had five moms. My parents separated when I was twelve, but we kept on being together for holidays. They just recently divorced, and we still all get together for holidays and special occasions.

My parents were both forty-four when I was born. They never really knew what was going on with me, like what I was into, and they couldn't relate to any of the music I was into or what I was thinking. There was a huge generation gap. My mother was very kind and loving and totally supportive, but there wasn't much communication between us. I'm a very vocal person and she's not, so sometimes there was friction because I'd get frustrated with her. She wouldn't really listen to me sometimes, and she didn't seem to be able to understand me. But she is so caring and giving in general, almost too sacrificial. I completely and totally respect her and love her a lot.

It's hard to describe my relationship with my father in the sense that he is really absorbed in himself, and he gets really neurotic and obsessive about things. When we talk he launches into a monologue about all of his activities, and I'm supposed to be the listener or the observer.

He'll ask me questions sometimes and then I'll respond, and then he'll turn the conversation back to himself. This is the way he is. That's why my mom couldn't stay with him, because he's so very self-centered.

My father was the boss in the house when I was a child. My mom was very subservient at that time. Once they separated, she started getting her life together and was much happier. He was a lab technician in a hospital, and he would work one night and be home the next. When he was home, that was his night of peace and quiet, and I couldn't have friends over. I couldn't be loud, and at the dinner table I couldn't talk. I couldn't make noises. I remember one time tracing my finger on the ketchup bottle, like on the little ridges, and he shouted "Stop that."

When I was younger, he used to spank me with the newspaper. It was nothing that really hurt, but it was an intimidation thing. He would get all mad, but I wasn't that scared of him. He did try to spend time with me, but it was more that he would incorporate me into his activities. He would suggest playing tennis and offer to teach me, but he's the one who liked tennis. He would never do anything that I wanted to do. Oh, I remember that once we saw a movie that I chose, but we didn't do that often. My dad's mom committed suicide when he was fifteen. She may have been manic-depressive. I think that's a lot why my dad is the way he is.

I don't know if I was happy at home as a child or not. It was mixed. I remember being really happy on the holidays because all my family was there, but then being severely disturbed the day after because they were all leaving. I was happy with my mom, but I remember being upset with my dad when I was younger.

But I was really unhappy in terms of school when I was growing up. I lived in a neighborhood where we sort of hung around in a group on the block. I was close friends with one or two of the girls in the group, but I was always the lowest on the totem pole. I had really low self-esteem within that group. I definitely felt unattractive and ugly growing up.

I remember being afraid to go to school sometimes in third grade because of some mean kids in my grade. Some days they would decide to pick on me and ignore me and push me, and do things like that. I would come home crying and tell my mom I didn't want to go to school. I didn't think my mom really understood, so I wouldn't talk about it much. Besides, I guess I felt there was nothing much she could do. I didn't want her calling any of their moms or anything like that.

I was a troublemaker in elementary school. I was the kid who was always being sent to the principal's office, mostly because I was really loud and I would talk back to the teachers when I got mad. My mom sent me to a therapist for a few sessions when I was nine, and all I remember is playing with toys there.

In junior high I started being more independent in terms of my friends and not trying so hard to conform. I shaved my head and wore different clothes. Shaving my head was definitely a rebellious thing. I thought of it as being more powerful or more defiant. I couldn't understand why some of the boys in my class who were also really defiant didn't become attracted to me. But I got so many remarks and evil criticisms after I did it that I felt even uglier than I had before.

One good thing happened that year—I made my first best friend. That next summer we made up an eating regimen. We were going to run around the track and go on a diet for the whole summer. That was the first time I started thinking much about what I ate.

My mom and sisters are all naturally thin and my dad's about average. I was chunky up until seven or eight, but then I thinned out a bit as I grew taller. I remember being called bean pole. I snacked a lot and my mom was always trying to get me to eat more food. She grew up right after the Depression and that affected her in that she liked to give us more food. We didn't have unhealthy food around like sweets or sugar cereals. I ate lots of cheese and fruit and meat and potato-type meals.

In eighth grade I started to develop and really fill out more. That's when I first started not liking the way I looked. I didn't feel that comfortable with my body. I would try to diet, like not eat much all day except some rice cakes. When I got tired of that, I would try some other strategy. Between diets I'd be normal for awhile.

By freshman year in high school, I was really afraid I was going to get fat. I was 5'7" and remember getting on the scale and hitting almost 150 pounds. So I went on a series of diets, but nothing worked. One night I ate a ton of pizza and I was so depressed. I was at a girl-friend's house, lying in bed, and suddenly something just clicked inside of me. I said to myself, "Tomorrow you are going to do it," and I did. The next day I started going to Weight Watchers. I stuck with it, and the weight slowly started coming off. When I hit the two-week mark I knew I was going to do it. I remember thinking that as soon as I lost weight I would be able to really live and be happy. And that did happen in the very beginning. The attention I received during this time was pretty outrageous—from the people at my school, from my teachers, from almost everyone I knew.

Up until this point the whole year had been really insecure for me. I was trying to get used to high school and I didn't know who my friends were. People were forming groups and making friends, and I didn't feel like I really had that. I had a weird crush on this older boy, a junior, who didn't even know me. Everyone found out about it and made fun of me. I was drunk at a party, I think, and told someone who spread it around. That was a hard, hard time for me. I didn't feel attractive at all, and I had never had a boyfriend.

When I started with Weight Watchers and lost some weight, it felt great when people started flooding me with comments. The way people changed toward me was amazing. I got a nickname, "Bones." It was sort of an esteemed name. I took it as people saying, "I am concerned about you but yet, wow, you are so skinny." The only thing anyone talked to me about was my weight. They wanted to know how I did it, and some people told me I was the first successful person they had ever known. So I kept on losing more weight.

I stayed on the meal plan for the first week of Weight Watchers. I never changed it. I just stayed there. It looked like a very healthy diet. I was eating the four food groups and salads, and that was much healthier than I had been eating before. So when school ended I was feeling more confident and really happy with all the attention I was getting. That summer I worked in a bakery and yet I never ate anything, which was something I really prided myself on. It was like the food was 1,000 miles away from me.

I was weighing myself every day, but it was a very abstract thing to me. I don't remember being that preoccupied with the weight. I would pinch myself to see where the fat was still on my body, and as long as there was extra skin even, I would say, "Okay, you still have more to go."

When I came back to school in tenth grade, everyone was stalking me because I was thinner than I had been before. It was this big deal. I weighed about 114 pounds and got nominated for Homecoming princess. I was upset because I felt like I didn't deserve it, and also I had never had that attention before, but I was also secretly thinking, "Wow, look at me!" I remember thinking weird things like the night of Homecoming that if I got it I would have to be this way forever. But I didn't win, and I'm glad because I'm so opposed to those types of things.

I was so thin that my bones were sticking out. I remember having a blackout one time. I was standing up and all of a sudden I fell backward onto the floor. I screamed and my sister came in. I jumped up and ran into my bed. I remember trying to laugh and deny there was a problem.

I couldn't sit on a chair for very long because it was too painful. One time I was stretching in front of my mirror in my bedroom and I caught sight of my whole rib cage. I mean it looked like my skeleton and it shocked me. My hair got really thin, though I didn't grow any hair on my body like some anorexics. My face was very, very pale and looked sunken in, and I had black smudges under my eyes.

So I knew things were weird, but I didn't know what to do. I was really isolated. People were starting to express concern now, but it was wrapped up in this jealous sort of compliment. I felt like I was guarding something and people wanted to take it away. My mom was cooking for me at the time, and I would accuse her of putting in an extra ounce of chicken or teaspoon of mayonnaise. I would get into these crazy yelling fits where I would accuse her of trying to make me fat. I got furious when I saw her reading books on eating disorders.

At the same time it was getting scary, it was also my identity, and I was very proud. It was such a protection. No one could take away my thinness; no one could say I was ugly or fat. It was such a powerful feeling. I don't think I have ever felt more powerful than at that time. Food meant nothing to me, and I would look at people eating and think how I didn't have to be weak like them.

But gradually I became tired all the time. I wasn't exercising at all because I was too tired. And I didn't want to go out with my group of friends. I never ate when I was out with them, and it became this big deal to try and get me to eat, so I stopped going. My bones started to stick out, my hair started falling out, and I was always cold. I remember freezing during hot days in the summer, and I would always wear my jacket. I just knew something was going on with my body. But, as I said, I was very alone and very guarded.

I remember how all my thoughts, slowly and progressively, were about food. I just slowly stopped thinking about dating guys or people I might be interested in. All I thought about was food. I wrote stories about food. I daydreamed about food. I was around food all the time, but I was starving. I remember that feeling of starvation. It was so intense that it permeated everything I did. I went to bed wanting to wake up to eat my little portions.

I let myself have a cup of fat-free cereal, ½ grapefruit, and a cup of nonfat milk for breakfast. For lunch I would have a piece of 40-calorie bread with one tablespoon Weight Watchers mayonnaise and an ounce or two of tuna, and an apple and carrot sticks. For dinner I would have a potato with nothing on it, and salad, and maybe a small bit of skinless chicken. Then there were times I would eat an extra apple, and I'd get really angry at myself and feel out of control.

I got really into cooking and I would have people come over. But of course I wouldn't eat anything, and I would pride myself on that. I would have people tell me what the food tasted like and describe it at length. I would send cookies off to people I knew in college. I constantly wanted to be around food.

Eventually, my mom took me to the doctor because I had to get a physical for athletics. Even though I was always tired, I wanted to participate in sports at school. The doctor told me that if I lost any more weight I would have to be hospitalized. I was maybe 110 pounds. That really affected me, the thought of having to go to the hospital. I was afraid of that for some reason.

I don't know what exactly triggered it, other than the fear of being hospitalized, but right after visiting the doctor I began eating fattening foods again. I guess I had reached the point where I was starving, and either something really bad was going to happen to me or I was going to have to eat. This was in the middle of tenth grade. But I just went crazy with food, and all of a sudden my nightmare was happening. I started eating so much. I tried to go back to my regimen, but then I would be so hungry. I ate things that I hadn't been able to eat. I would tell myself that just this one day I'd go off my diet, and eat and taste as much as I could before I'd go back to it. But on the days I was trying to be strict, I would get home after school and start to eat just one cookie and I would just keep on eating. I mean, amazing amounts of food like a box of cookies and a whole pizza. I definitely ate way past the limit my little stomach could possibly take at that time. My system was so backed up that I just felt like I was exploding.

I would try to purge, but sometimes I couldn't do it. It was hard to make myself gag. I tried laxatives just once and that didn't really work. My mom found out about it and it became too complicated. So usually I would go to bed just so distraught. I was the most depressed I've ever been. Gradually I gained all the weight back, plus more. I got up to around 160 pounds. That summer I remember just sitting home and eating. That's all I would do. I would think how fat and ugly I was and get really, really upset at myself. One day I was so depressed that I ran out of the house and hid in a neighbor's driveway. I was at such a low point I just wanted to die. I didn't want to talk to my mom about it because I didn't feel that close to her, but I called one of her friends. She was inspiring and supportive, and after that I went on another diet.

This time I went to the Weight Watcher meetings, which I hadn't done before. I wanted to lose weight and psychologically know how to deal with it. My goal was reasonable for my bone structure—130 pounds. I lost about seven pounds really quickly, and began getting attention again for losing weight. I slowly got back into the same thing. I got way down and was really skinny again for about six months. But then I reached a point where I was so hungry that I went berserk again. It terrified me to be in that horrible space where I felt like I was starving. So I started eating and the whole cycle started up again. I got really depressed. I stayed home, except for going to school, and wore really baggy clothing. I wore more fitting clothing when I was thinner. But when I was bigger I would just wear my sweats, just completely de-sexualize myself. I didn't exercise and would go five days without taking a shower or washing my hair. When I was thinner I took a shower every day.

My close friends were still my close friends, but it wasn't like they were concerned about me anymore. No one really talked about my weight, and I just felt like a failure. When I was thin they would ask me how I did it, what to do, because they were all dieting too. Two friends were really supportive when I started getting really thin. They told me I didn't look very good instead of complimenting me like everyone else did. They would tell me I didn't have the energy I used to have. I had been a gregarious, lively person, but all that went away. But when I gained all the weight back, all my friends avoided the subject, so no one knew what I was going through.

One of my teachers tried to help when I got too thin. She told me that she had been anorexic, and she described what it had been like for her. What she said fit into how I was feeling, though I had never thought of myself as anorexic before. We had some good talks, and she always sort of looked out for me. But when I gained the weight back, I thought that I didn't deserve her attention anymore. We still had contact, but not as much. I didn't feel that I could talk to her anymore because she was obviously still thinner. She hadn't ballooned out like me. I was ashamed. I was really ashamed that I lost the control.

During all this time, from junior high and all throughout high school, I got straight A's. School was the one thing I would prioritize above all else. I was just determined. It was my identity to be the straight A student. My parents were happy for me, proud of me, but they didn't push me to do this or reward me. I knew I could work hard, but I didn't think I was very intelligent. Even though I was proud of myself, I felt that anyone else could also do this well, too, if they just worked hard.

The summer between my junior and senior year I went to France and lived with a family there for two months. One of my sisters urged me to go and helped me financially. It was really good for me. I was still stressed about my weight, but I walked all over and got a lot of exercise. I traveled and improved my French, and it was really a wonderful experience. I got out of my depression, and thinking about my weight and food every single minute, because there was so much to see and do. I just naturally lost weight without even trying. I came back to school looking healthy and tan. People were more responsive to me again. They admired me for going to France and were more interested in me. I felt great and wore clothes that were more sexual. A lot of guys in my class said they'd never seen me look greater. I felt more attractive and looked forward to having a good senior year.

But again I started eating out of control. I was really big in my senior year, and I was really depressed. I felt really ugly and horrible, and then I graduated. So my high school career was just a period of ups and downs. At the time I felt like my only disorder was my thinness. I didn't see my compulsive overeating or my being so overweight as being part of the illness.

Now, as I look back, I wonder about how an earlier incident affected me. When I was younger, I remember feeling sexual. I was interested in boys when I was about eight years old. I remember feeling ashamed because I experimented with one boy in the neighborhood, and my mom and some neighbors found out. We just kissed, but it became this very shameful thing.

Then, when I was nine, I was interested in a boy who was a year older. One night a bunch of us slept in a tent in a neighbor's backyard. One of my sisters was there, and so was my dad. But when everyone was sleeping, this boy touched me in places I didn't want to be touched. That was the first sexual experience I ever had, and I was disgusted by it. I don't even know what to label it. I guess he molested me. He touched me on my breasts and in my genital area and kept trying to kiss me. He was very experienced, and told me he had sex with some older girls and women. I was just sort of floored and didn't know what to do. I moved far away from him, and then he stopped. I felt so powerless and gross. I remember feeling really horrible about it for a long time.

After that experience I ceased having sexual feelings. I never had a boyfriend in junior high or high school. I had no sexual experience, so I felt very asexual. I think that any time boys became interested in me I felt very threatened and used food to escape from the situation. I made myself either so sick or so unattractive that everyone left me alone.

College was the greatest thing that has ever happened to me. When I started I was still feeling very fat and depressed. But I met women who were big, who were strong, who didn't shave or conform to any beauty norm. I made good friends who respected me for my intelligence and my sense of humor. They didn't care about my looks or how good I was at partying. For the first time I had friends who were good people, loving people. They knew how to prioritize friendship, so that their boyfriends didn't always come first before their women friends. It was just the greatest thing to feel so accepted for who I was. I really grew and started to love myself.

In my mind I still wanted to lose weight, but I let myself eat whatever I wanted for the first time without worrying about it. I walked all over and got exercise, and became healthier. That lasted my freshman year and into sophomore year.

Then I became interested in Jake. I didn't know if he felt the same way about me. All the old insecurities came up, like how could anyone ever like me, and how uncomfortable the sexual realm was for me. I started starving myself again because I figured there was no way he was going to be interested in me unless I was thin. I lost a lot of weight and I felt more attractive. But then I couldn't stop myself from losing more and more weight. I felt so out of control, so depressed that it was happening again, when I thought I was over that. I heard the voices again, the things I was feeling, telling me, "You can do it. You can lose all this weight." I had thought I was a feminist and stronger than that by now, but all of a sudden I rocketed back into this weird state.

That lasted just a few months this time. Jake, as it turned out, was interested in me before I even lost all the weight. We just were both so insecure in the beginning. We got together and it was great. We thought we were so in love, and he was really supportive. He was the first person I had a sexual relationship with. It wasn't a very good one at first, though. I was gradually gaining back all the weight and felt devastated about it. Deep down I still thought he would probably like me more if I was thinner. At first, I felt ashamed and uncomfortable about my body and couldn't really enjoy sex with him. But we could talk about my feelings, and that helped because he was always so reassuring. I'm still with him. It's been over two years and now it's great. It's been the first time I have ever felt beautiful or at all sexual.

A few things have helped me get over my eating disorder. Being around my friends who really love me for who I am, that's important. Being around people who want to enjoy food and who love food.

Dancing really helps—being able to release tension and have fun with my friends. We go dancing one or two nights a week. When I'm dancing I feel really one with my body and just happy. It helps to have a supportive boyfriend who thinks I'm attractive even if I sometimes think I'm too big.

I never really got professional help, although it was something I wanted to do. I didn't have the money, and I didn't think I needed help unless I was really thin. I didn't know that I should have gone when I felt so fat. It was this weird thing—I felt like I didn't have an eating disorder, I was just fat again. On campus, we're just allowed eight free counseling sessions and that didn't appeal to me. I wanted someone I could see continually.

One of the best things that I did was get involved with a group on campus called Body Awareness. It's actually an accredited course. It's a group of women and a few men who developed a curriculum to go into schools, from elementary to high school, and talk about body awareness and eating disorders. When I first heard about it, I thought I have to do this program because it was the first time I could take all my experience and put it into something positive. The first time I ever told my story was during one of our training sessions. It really affected everyone there. People came up and told me such beautiful things—that I was so powerful, that my story really had meaning. They totally understood **and** validated what I said. This class was a channel for me. I realized how many people go through an eating disorder, and that I could still be powerful even if this was my downfall.

It's meant so much to me on so many different levels. I love talking to kids, and sharing my story with them. It's such a good feeling to know I'm helping even just one person who's listening to what I have to say. And it helps me feel powerful because now I'm helping train new people and put together new materials. I see myself working in this field, in education or social work, helping educate women about body image issues.

I eat very well now. I'm very knowledgeable and have tons of cook-books. I am really into cooking, for the taste and for the community feeling. I live in a house off-campus and my roommates and I take turns cooking. There are still times where I'll overeat, but I can accept it and am generally okay with it.

I still have occasional fat attacks, as we call them in our body aware-ness class. I'll wake up and notice my body and the fat on my body. I'll get the same feeling I used to get when I stepped on the scale, like, oh my God, I am going to balloon out. But I have learned to calm myself down, and that feeling eventually goes away. I see it as just a cycle, and that I am going to have those off days. Because most of the time I am fine with my body and I think it is beautiful. I have stopped wearing only baggy clothes. I'm 5'9" now, and weigh somewhere between 150–160 pounds. But I don't weigh myself anymore. If my clothes are start-ing to feel too tight, I just try to cut back a little or exercise more.

It helps that there are so many things I am involved in. I am doing an internship, working with people recovering from drugs and alcohol. There are things I'm doing that are very powerful. My weight isn't my only security. I feel intelligent, I feel I am doing well in school, I love the people I live with, I love a lot of what I'm doing. I try to give myself affirmations, tell myself good things. So I feel really positive about myself most of the time now.

My advice for others is to try to invest yourself in other things, to find security in other things besides your body. Try to appreciate your body for the way it can function and how you can use it, not just for how it looks. It helps to read books and educate yourself about eating disorders. Definitely surround yourself with people who love you and who aren't going to be concerned with beauty and thinness and things like that. Try to concentrate on your health and feeling good physically too. Get help if you can afford it or join a group. It's important to talk about it and be understood, so that you don't have to be ashamed of having this problem.

4

NANCY

Nancy is a 48-year-old married mother of two. She teaches dance and aerobics, and is a certified personal trainer. She struggled with bulimia, on and off, for more than twenty-two years. Nancy has been symptom-free for eight years.

I grew up in a large family of seven children in a suburb outside of San Francisco. My dad is a doctor, a heart specialist, and my mom was a homemaker. Then she went back to school and became an artist. I was the sixth of seven children. I had three older brothers, two older sisters, then me, and a little brother who was five years younger. My mom was either breast-feeding or pregnant for about nine years straight. I got along great with my two sisters, but I didn't know my older brothers all that well since they were so much older.

My relationship with my parents was wonderful. It was really busy in the house, and I think my sisters took more care of me than my parents did. I love my parents, and we still have a really good relationship. I think I had a normal upbringing. We had a housekeeper throughout my childhood who would always have food for the neighborhood kids to eat when they came over. We were leniently raised, but not spoiled, I don't think. My mom loved children and has always been a really maternal person. Anybody who needed someplace to play or hang out could always come to our house. The neighbors always thought we were too noisy and too many cars were around, but we were happy for the most part.

When I think back to how my eating disorder started, there are a few things I remember. One thing that happened all the time was that my mom was always, always complaining about her weight. She would always say, "Oh, I'm so fat, I can't eat that"—and this was before eating disorders were really known. She was always trying to chew Trident gum or doing something so she wouldn't eat. And we were very conscious of this. One of my sisters was a heavy girl, but I was born with a really fast metabolism and was always really skinny from the time I was little. After dinner my parents would always make me eat the leftovers, or if there was one more glass of milk, they'd say, "Oh, Nancy should have it. She hasn't had enough to eat." One scary thing I remember was when I was about fourteen and walking down the hall at school, and my thighs rubbed together. It scared me because I realized that I was either getting fat or I was turning into a woman.

When I was around eleven or twelve, I was sexually attacked. All I can remember is being pulled into a tent when my family was hiking up a local mountain. I had become a little separated from them. Some guy pulled his pants down and forced his penis into my mouth. So I think there was quite some fear in becoming a woman. I didn't tell anyone. I just totally put that out of my mind. And then sometime around the time when I was seventeen, I went to get my hair done and the owner of the hairdressing salon took me into the back and forced me into the same situation. So there was always a fear of growing into a woman. I actually forgot about both these incidents until they came back to me when I was about thirty-three and in therapy.

I was a pretty little teenager, and I was always thin and I was always blonde. But my brothers' friends would always look at me, and I was afraid that if I allowed myself to be pretty that I'd get into trouble. That's why I loved going to dance classes, because it was a relief to be allowed to be pretty and beautiful in the dance studio. It was okay there. But otherwise, when I was home or anywhere else, it was really quite a scary thing because I might bring on sexual confrontations or something.

I started taking dance when I was thirteen or fourteen, but didn't seriously start dancing until I was sixteen. There was always somebody in class that I admired greatly, that was beautiful or whom I wanted to be, and I never had enough confidence in myself. But I knew there was something in it that was really releasing for me. And I just loved it. But it was funny; whenever I got to the point where I could have gone to a really professional dance camp or something like that, I would always do something to foul myself up so that I wouldn't actually be successful. I don't know what it was. But eventually I got to dance in San Francisco in a cabaret-like show. We performed with a local comedienne and pretty soon the crowds got packed.

I started being bulimic when I was seventeen. Everybody in the dance world was so obsessed with being thin. You would either throw up, or you wouldn't eat, or you would take drugs, or smoke, or whatever it was. And so that became the norm. The people I admired in class had certain physiques, and I would think if I had that physique I'd be able to dance like them. I wanted to be somebody else and look like somebody else, and I thought it was thinness that made them great. I never really got there because, of course, you cannot attain that ability unless you love yourself. It was not until years later that I was able to love myself, in my thirties, and by then I had become a better dancer.

One of the dancers I admired most was named Carol. I just thought she was the greatest thing in the world. I knew if she wasn't dancing, or was hurt, or couldn't take class, that she wouldn't eat. She would skip all her meals and then maybe have a drink at night. In fact I remember one time going into a bar and seeing her there. I said something like, "Oh, aren't you eating?" She said, "Oh no, I'm not going to eat. I can't take class because I hurt my foot. So I'm not eating." I thought, "Oh my God, how can she not eat? It's amazing. Where does she get that willpower and that strength? I need to be like her."

One day I threw up and realized how easy it was. I remember going home with giant amounts of cake and ice cream, and letting myself eat all I wanted because I'd found a way to control myself. When I binged, I would always have sweets. In the beginning, I only did it once in awhile, kind of as an experiment. It wasn't really something I thought about much.

When I think back, I realize that I was surrounded by people concerned about their weight at that time. And though my dad always told me how smart I was and would call me "pretty girl," he was a very thin man and was always conscious about gaining weight. He's in medicine, and he always believed that you were healthier if you were thinner. And my mom was always trying to lose weight, so there was a weight issue there. My dad expected us girls to be beautiful and marry well. I used to be afraid my sisters wouldn't like me because he didn't call them "pretty girl," only me. He would make comments to my sister who was heavy, kind of make her feel bad about the way she looked, and she wouldn't say anything. My sister has gotten quite heavy in the last ten years, and to this day he will say stuff about it to her. Only now she tells him to shut up.

My dancing career took off when a choreographer saw our act and hired us to dance with a well-known rock band. The band got quite famous for awhile. We toured in Europe four times and around the United States. I wasn't bulimic during this time because I was so involved in drinking and drugs, and was very thin because of all that. The lead guitarist, Don, and I had a great explosive relationship, very exciting—drugs, and rock and roll, and all that kind of stuff. We did cocaine, mostly, and drank a lot. After a few years, I got to the point where I couldn't stand the lifestyle anymore. I was realizing it was basically going to kill me, and I was getting really depressed. I got pregnant at twenty-five, hoping that would help me get out of that cycle and it did. Don and I got married when I was three months pregnant. Then, all of a sudden, I had a kid and had to stay at home and could not go on tour.

When I was pregnant, I tried really hard not to do drugs and drink. But after the baby, the only way Don and I could connect when he came home was by doing drugs or going out partying. I would have this life when he was away that was very normal and kind of nice, though I missed dancing and the excitement. Then he would come home, and everything would turn upside down again, and fall back in the hole again. We started smoking opium. That was pretty addictive and got pretty scary.

I got pregnant again when our first child, Nick, was less than a year old. This time, I actually did cocaine a couple of times, and smoked opium once or twice when I was pregnant. I also became bulimic again. I remember visiting the band when they were doing a video at a recording studio in London during this time. The choreographer came up to me and said something about how he could put a glass on my hip, signifying that I had gained so much weight in my hips. I remember being just absolutely devastated by him saying that. I thought I should not be getting fat, even if I was pregnant. And that here was this man I admired so much, who could make all the difference in the world to me. I was really missing dancing with the band and all the excitement. I thought maybe I'd be able to dance again if I did exactly what he said, that maybe he would hire me back after the baby. And maybe the way to do that was to be thin, whether I was pregnant or not. I remember wanting to be normal like everyone else. In other words, being pregnant meant I was fat, and so I was not normal.

My pregnancy with my daughter, Christine, was horrible, unhealthy, and depressing. I look at the pictures now and it was like a whole other person. I was still bingeing and purging, and I was really sick. I was way underweight, and my doctor put me into the hospital at seven months because I was having way too many problems. After Christine was born, I realized I needed help. It wasn't just bulimia I was worried about; it was also drugs and alcohol. Life was getting pretty dangerous once again. I persuaded Don to move back near my parents so I'd have their help while he was away. But he started doing more drugs, as I was trying to do less, and we just fought all the time. I thought he was getting really distant and that he was having other relationships. It was just a terribly, terribly lonely time, and I was in a lot of pain.

After Christine was born, I went back to work teaching dance classes at night. That was too hard with the kids, though, so I found a job teaching aerobics during the day. It gave me a little bit of freedom and made me feel like I was actually doing something. Oddly enough, my favorite thing really was being with the kids and being at home. But there was a sadness to it because it was not a family situation or a happy married situation. So I think the sadness made me want to go off and have a profession to still be who I was.

During this time drinking became a really big problem for me because I quit taking drugs. I still had bulimia, but I was so depressed and in so much pain that drinking wine became my mainstay. Don was off having affairs, and he lied to me about it in front of the therapist we were seeing. I felt just completely worthless.

I was being bulimic every day, sometimes as much as five times a day. I held breakfast down, but not lunch or dinner. My worst times were in the late afternoons. I think something that triggered it was nightfall, because I think the transitions between day and night were always very scary for me. I hated twilight and I would get morbidly depressed at this time of day. I usually ate dinner, but about a half hour later I would go and binge and purge. I would always wake up in the middle of the night and eat again, kind of in my sleep, and then I would go back to sleep. My body was probably starving at this point. I started tying the refrigerator closed at night because I thought this might wake me up before I would eat, but that didn't work.

So not only was I hung over the next day, but I also felt sick from the bulimia. One of the biggest problems I had was living in "now." I would never remember how horrible I felt the day after drinking and bingeing and purging. I only lived for right now, today, so I had to have quick fixes. I always felt too fat, and I didn't know how to tell myself, "If you really want to lose weight, you can do it slowly over two to three months."

This was such an awful period for me. I had stomachaches. I had horrible gas. It was embarrassing. I couldn't go out sometimes if I had three to four days of bad bulimic episodes. My stomach was swollen all the time, and my esophagus hurt all the time when I swallowed. At first I didn't notice that my teeth were bad. I had gone to a bulimia meeting at Overeaters Anonymous and a woman said to wash your mouth out with baking soda so your teeth don't get ruined. When I finally went to the dentist he asked me if I had an eating disorder and I said, "No."

My gums receded, and they became extremely sensitive. I would have to use Sensodyne toothpaste. I think that the last few years that I was really bad off, I used baking soda so much that I didn't have as much damage as I could have. And I think it probably even saved my esophagus and my stomach. I have a lot of fillings, and my teeth at the root were horrible. I have had seven root canals, so seven of my teeth have died. I am sure it was because of the bulimia, no doubt in my mind.

Through all of this, I didn't care to live basically, but I loved my kids so much that I couldn't let myself die. There were several times when I really almost died, and my parents would come over and make me eat. At one point I weighed about 98 pounds—I'm normally about 130 pounds—and my parents just stuck with me and helped me through it. They didn't know I had an eating disorder the first few years. They just thought I wasn't able to take good care of myself.

Because of his drug problem, Don was in really bad straits and was not able to do anything financially. So I did not get any money from him, but my parents helped me consistently every month. Don and I tried for two years, off and on, to make the relationship work again, but it wouldn't. There was a lot of lying in our marriage because he was having affairs, and then I started having them too because I was so vindictive. I don't think I made a mistake in marrying Don when I did, but doing drugs and all the stuff we did in our relationship was a mistake.

When I was thirty-two, we got divorced. It seems so young to me now, but then I was worried about being old and not meeting anyone. Being a single mother and divorced, I think I put pressure on myself to stay thin and "beautiful," so I could eventually remarry and be taken care of. And I think I started putting emphasis on that being important if I wanted to get a man, because it was going to be hard since I was divorced with two kids.

I saw a few therapists during these years, paid for by my parents, but I only told one of them I had an eating disorder. I remember getting up the nerve to tell him, and he said, "Oh I do that, too. I get a beautiful porcelain dish and put candles all around, and then I throw up." I thought to myself, he really was lying to me, that he doesn't do that, and that he doesn't really have any idea what I am talking about. What he may have been trying to say, in a really weird kind of way, was that it was okay to be throwing up. But it wasn't okay with me, so having it be okay with him was not going to make it any better for me. I kept wanting to get at the root of what was bugging me so I could just take care of it. Either I wasn't ready to get better or that wasn't the right therapy for me.

Looking back, I can see some things I did which made me feel awful about myself. A few years after the first sexual attack, I became pretty promiscuous. I had sex for the first time when I was fourteen. Right before my fifteenth birthday, I got pregnant and had an abortion. There was a definite feeling that I owed it to men to have sex with them, because I led them to believe that I liked them, or because they made me think I turned them on. Since I had already been abused and I wasn't really worthwhile anyway, what was there to lose? I think it was like covering up pain, trying to have fun, and to find something that felt good.

I used to steal, but not in a conscious way. I wouldn't go into Macy's and steal bras and stuff, but I would "accidentally" walk out of a store with a pair of sunglasses on my head. I would take stuff home from work all the time. When I had a job I hated, working at a health club, I wanted to quit, but got fired instead. That made me so mad that, before I left, I took three-hole punchers, and staplers, and whatever I could take. I was so vindictive and angry at them because I was not going to have this job, even though I didn't even want the job. Another time, I was shopping and didn't realize I hadn't been charged for a fan until I got home. But I didn't take it back because I hadn't consciously walked off with it. I had been so dishonest and quiet about my behavior for so many years that I literally didn't know how to be honest.

My parents raised me that it was important not to lie, so there was a certain boundary that I would not cross. But if it was about being bulimic I could lie about that, and if it was about my marriage, which was a mess anyway, I could certainly lie about that. When I finally told my parents and Don about the bulimia, after I'd gotten the divorce, it was the beginning of my recovery.

What really helped me recover was the intense love I had for my kids. I just had to do it for them. I almost feel like I recovered because of them and not because of myself, although I hate to say that because I don't want people who don't have kids not to want to recover. I knew if I could love somebody as much as I loved them that I could be a good person. And I knew I was a good mother. I think that being a mother gave me the one thing in life that I knew I could do well. Even if I didn't think I was dancing well, or cleaning house well, or cooking well, I knew I was a good mother. That gave me a positive reason for trying to help myself. I started spending more time at home with them, and some days I would not be bulimic.

Around this time I started working with a wonderful therapist named Connie. She helped me figure out all the reasons I didn't love myself or even like myself, going back to when I was first sexually attacked. I call the sexual harassment experiences rapes, although they were not physically penetrating.

When I met Connie I had been having horrible, horrible nightmares. They were just excruciating. One was where I walked into the driveway of my house and there were two Japanese warriors fighting. I am pretty sure they were me, the two Nancy's—the good Nancy and the bad Nancy. One of them cut off the head of the other, and the head went spinning through the air, with blood flying everywhere. It is really hard to describe how horrible it was. I wasn't sure when I was talking to Connie whether it was the good one or the bad one who died, and she would help me find the words to describe how I was feeling.

Another dream that I had a lot while I was bulimic, was being in a cabin, lying on a plank floor. Underneath the floor was all this vomit, and it was filled with snakes. They would be coming up through the planks of the floor, trying to get me. I am terrified of snakes. I hate snakes, and I would always have snake dreams when I was at the worst of my bulimia. I would also have these horrible dreams about toilets and vomit and excrement. In therapy, I would cry when I talked about these dreams, and the words would just pour out. I was able to do the most unbelievable work with my therapist.

Little by little, there would be a week, and then a month, that I would not be bulimic. Then there were two months, then three months, and then there was literally a six-month period. It got to the point where I felt like I had some control over it, though I hate to say that because it was such a controlling thing. What was interesting was that, for the first time, I was paying for therapy myself instead of having my parents pay for it.

One thing I used to do was have a ribbon in my bathroom—a long, pink ribbon from a present—and I had stars, because I used to do star projects with the children when they were young. Every day, if I was good and didn't drink or wasn't bulimic, I would give myself a star. If it wasn't a good day, I'd put a circle written in pen which didn't look very pretty on the ribbon. So I started watching my progression of the stars on this ribbon, and I wanted to see more stars. It also helped me remember the next day how I had been the day before. It was a visual way to see some progress.

Right after the divorce I had a couple of boyfriends, and then I met Jeff who I'm married to now. We met at the health club where I worked before I got fired, and actually I was drinking a lot at that time. We dated for three years, and I don't know why he never said anything to me about my drinking. Maybe he just saw something beneath all the problems, I don't know. I was definitely getting better at that time, and I was working with Connie. I fell in love with him, and I was terrified of going back into the horrible life I'd had. I remember driving home from work one day and thinking to myself, "Oh my God, I am actually happy." I had a happy feeling, and I did not even know what it was at first. I didn't remember being happy for years and years. I felt there was actually good happening in my life, and it was unbelievable.

Well, shortly after I had that good feeling that day, his parents talked him into breaking up with me because I had been married and had two kids. We had an enormous break-up, and it was horrible and devastating. I came out of it okay though, after a couple of weeks, but he didn't. He realized he really loved me, and that his parents had been wrong. We got married in 1991, and I was still bulimic at the time. I hadn't told Jeff about my eating disorder at all because I was afraid he wouldn't want me if he knew. I was at the point where I'd go three months or six months without doing it, and I would think I was over it, but then I would have an episode. I finally broke down one day when I was sitting in the bedroom. He came in and asked me why I was so upset. I told him I had an eating disorder, and he needed to know about it, but that I was sure I was going to lose him. I was expecting him to have a big reaction, like holding onto my ankles and saying, "Oh my God, what should we do?" But he just told me it was no big deal and that I should take care of it. So I went about taking care of it.

I still had my drinking to deal with, too, since I would still get really drunk at times. I went to AA and tried to quit drinking completely, but what happened instead was that I started drinking less and less. Going to AA did not work for me. I just didn't relate to anybody in there for some reason. I guess the same way I recovered with bulimia worked with my problem with alcohol. I just felt that I had to do it, and it slowly became controllable. Still, to this day I am totally careful. I will have one or two glasses of wine, but if I get the feeling of getting outside myself, that scares me, and I will stop drinking.

I stopped smoking the same way, by gradually cutting down. I smoked on and off, from the time I met Don when I was about twenty years old, until about the same time I quit being bulimic. I never smoked unless I was drinking or doing drugs, so I was a weekend or night smoker. Christine, my daughter, hated smoke and hated seeing me smoke. I know I did not stop because of her, but she was a big influence. I loved her, and I wanted to be able to be a good example for her. I just tried to smoke less and less, and I would praise myself if it was two days apart, or then three days apart. Now I haven't smoked in over eight years.

A few months after I recovered from bulimia, Connie put me on Prozac. It took her a long time to convince me to do it. I think that one reason was that it had been so hard for me to get off drugs, and I just could not stand the thought of being on drugs again. It was terrifying to me, and I did not want to be dependent on anything again. It was kind of funny that, out of all these therapists that I went to, nobody treated me for depression. There is schizophrenia on both my mother's side of the family and on my father's side. My father's sister was diagnosed with schizophrenia when she was sixteen, and was in and out of institutions her whole life before she died in her forties. I'm actually named after her. On my mother's side, two of her sisters and some of their children, my cousins, were diagnosed with either depression, manic-depression, or schizophrenia.

I am still taking Prozac, but only a low dose of it. It lessens my sexual drive which I do not like at all. But it helps me avoid feeling as desperate as I used to, where I would go into a black hole and cry for hours, feeling depression washing into my body. Now, that desperation still comes in at times and I can feel it, but I can handle it better.

Gradually, I got less compulsive about eating and what I would eat. When I was bulimic, I was very obsessive about not eating fat. Let me tell you, there is nothing worse than having no fat in your diet at all, especially when you are exercising a lot. I used to count my calories and my fat grams. I kept books on what I ate during the day, why I ate it, and when I threw up. Now, I will eat fat, and I don't count anything anymore. I know now that when I eat fat and butter and nuts and chocolate I will feel better. I think, because of my body type, I probably wouldn't have ever gained weight anyway, so what I put myself through is really sad.

I also used to be compulsive about taking vitamins, even when I was at my worst bulimia. I figured I'd try to do something good for myself, even when I was doing something bad. But I overdosed on vitamin A twice. I was drinking carrot juice every day and taking vitamin A supplements and beta-carotene. I became completely fatigued to the point where I could not move. Finally I went to a doctor who diagnosed the problem. I still take vitamins and supplements, but am careful to stay within the recommended amounts.

Another way that I've changed is in my exercise patterns. I teach dance classes and aerobics classes at a local health club, and am a certified personal trainer. I used to do all my classes with everybody all the time. I guess I was compulsively exercising. Now I limit my exercise to no more than one hour a day at most, and I will actually teach without doing the actual exercise, or will just do it minimally. My newly found love is yoga. I think that helps me to slow down and concentrate more.

I am looking for ways to make myself happier and more content. The biggest thing for me is to slow down. I think the first few minutes of my slowing down are always really hard. Contentment always seems to come after about twenty to thirty minutes of putting my feet up, maybe reading, and just stopping. Then I can put things into perspective. But if I am going fast and there is a lot to do, if I have a lot of stress and worries, then I am miserable. I become so scattered that I can't figure out what is making me feel stressed and unhappy.

Sometimes, though, I think I'm happier when I am working more and don't have as much time to sit with myself. I can still get pretty darn miserable, especially in the winter. I know I am very affected by the seasons and light.

Discontentment is something that still comes at me from every corner sometimes, and it's still a continuous struggle. I think I will always have the sense of not actually being where I want to be. Speaking positively to myself helps because I tend to be a negative figure to myself. When I start telling myself, "You did not do this" or "You did that" or "You're not this or not that," I will just stop myself. Instead I'll repeat something like "I am beautiful, I am good, I love life, I am happy" over and over again for a half hour or so, and somehow it works.

It helps if I recognize when I am really tired because that's often when my discontentment sets in. I have a lot of physical problems that tire me out. I have had spinal stenosis in two places from a car accident when I was seventeen. And I had Lyme disease for an entire year before it was diagnosed. I was told that, because it wasn't treated for so long, it can be neurologically damaging for life. When I teach too many classes or get really stressed, my immune system breaks down. I will get a rash and get sick, so I have to be really careful.

I have become a lot more accepting of myself, in the way I look, or the things I say. But it is continuous work. I'm a kind of loud, "jump-in-with-both feet" kind of person, which used to cause me a lot of embarrassment. But now I think that's just the way I am, and I don't feel bad about it. I am much more loving outwardly than I was before, and I think that has helped a lot. I used to be critical and condescending of other people, but now I am much more accepting of everybody else, as well as myself.

My kids' father, Don, and I are great friends now. He's been straight for fifteen years, I'm happy to say. He is a great dad, and we love him completely. I have a close relationship with Jeff and my kids, and that, of course, makes me happy. Being honest with all of them has helped tremendously. I am calmer and able to appreciate what I have.

5

MICHAEL

Michael is a 53-year-old social worker. He struggled with obesity and compulsive overeating from childhood until age thirty-eight.

I grew up in an Irish-Catholic, Portuguese, alcoholic family. I found out my mother was alcoholic when I was nineteen, and I always knew my father drank too much. I was the youngest of three boys, the baby of the family, the apple of my mother's eye. My childhood was in the suburbs of Los Angeles, in a mostly Catholic neighborhood where there were more lushes than you could believe. Most of the women were drinking at ten in the morning, and the men that were around were always hitting the booze.

My main problem though, which continued for so much of my life, was with food. I remember being about seven or eight and seeing a picture of myself, but not recognizing myself because I was so fat. I had this image, until then, of being a regular-size kid, so it was a shock to see what I really looked like. I tried to convince everybody that it was somebody else. I know from my birth certificate I was around seven pounds at birth, so I was thin then. But from then on I have not had any memories of being thin in size, except when I took amphetamines back in the diet pill days, and then I was thin for a big twenty seconds. When I stopped taking them, I went right back up.

My father was fat, and one of my brothers was fat, but I was always the morbidly obese one. I remember being 200 pounds as a kid at 5'6", and later, as an adult, I weighed over 300 pounds. I went to Catholic schools, and in terms of education, I was very successful in school until the fourth grade. My teacher, Sister Irene, who was one of the crueler nuns, made fun of my weight in front of the class. I was really hurt by it. I told my parents, but they just shined it on and didn't do anything about it. I went downhill from then on, from being an A student to getting C's. I had a D-average in high school.

We always had large meals when I was growing up, and we always had dessert. We ate way too much food. Food was a big deal in my house. My mother cooked huge amounts of food, and we could stuff ourselves with as much as we wanted. My mother was big on red meat and then turning it into casseroles with noodles and gravy. Our refrigerator was always loaded with food which we could eat anytime we wanted. I remember being about nine or ten and eating so much spaghetti and raviolis to the point of being sick. I remember having stomach aches and crying all night long. Then I'd have that compulsive overeating kind of illness afterward. I'd have a taste in my mouth, like rotten eggs, and have ongoing nausea. Nobody ever said too much about it. They noticed I was feeling ill, but I don't think anybody knew what to do. They were too busy with their own lives. I just kind of figured that was what everybody did when they ate.

My mother put me on a diet once, something she read about in one of the women's magazines. It was a shake kind of thing that was supposed to substitute for some meals. I did lose weight with those drinks, but of course I put it back on as soon as I stopped. In eighth grade, I went into see the school nurse who lectured me about proper nutrition and said I needed to say no to food. But by then, even if I wanted to stop eating so much, I never could, no matter what I did. I would lose weight but never lose enough. Then I'd always gain it right back, and some more on top of it.

All the families in our neighborhood had a charge account at a tiny little grocery store down the hill. The owner would let families run up a tab and pay their accounts at the end of the month. So I would buy stuff that looked like it was for dinner, and sign off for it. I also would buy the family-size packages of M&M's and eat one of those each day after school. I guess my mother never checked what was on the bill; she just paid it.

I was obese, but at the same time I was a tough kid. I was active in sports and leadership activities, so I wasn't labeled "the fat kid." People knew if they teased me I would probably hit them, and I hit pretty hard. I was a scrapper because I had all this fear and rage from the way my father was with me. If anyone messed with me, I would just keep going and going.

My father was definitely king of the house. He was the breadwinner and earned all of the money. You did not mess with him. If you did, you would be on the losing end. He was a belt kind of guy. He didn't hesitate to drag out the belt if he thought we had gone too far. I learned to lie and duck and get sneaky because I was afraid of him. He would come home from work at night, after stopping off for a few drinks at the bar, and walk into the kitchen where my mother would do the Ozzie and Harriet housewife bit. He would reach under the table and bring out a bottle of Imperial Whiskey and have two big shots. He'd eat dinner and then proceed to have a couple of drinks afterward. He liked his booze. The other side of him was very successful, and driven, and family-oriented.

My mom took care of the house, so there was a stereotypical division of roles. She was kind of poetic and shy. She was withdrawn and had very few friends. She was an avid reader, and there were books all over the house. I was her favorite, the chosen one, and the boundaries between us were unclear. I was the repository of my mom's affection, and she was mine. It was very confusing to me as a kid. It was a very oedipal relationship. My mother had a number of heart attacks when I was seven and eight years old, so there was a lot of worry about her. She insisted I learn to cook then, so my dad could come home to a good home-cooked meal.

The rules were very rigid in our family, and the primary mode of control was shame. My parents were both loving, but very focused on themselves and their own issues and problems. Appearances were very important to them. There were many rules where food was concerned. We ate only with sterling silverware, and food had to be handled in the proper way. There was a lot of middle-class Irish pretentiousness. I wanted so much to believe we were all happy and would grow up happily ever after, so it was quite disappointing that life wasn't like that.

I got self-conscious about my weight when I started high school. I was not about to get naked in gym class. So I sat all through high school and watched sports that I would have liked to have participated in. I would have done the sports, but when the teacher kept bugging me to take a shower, I said no, and the school didn't do anything.

During this time I often drank like a fish. I had my first drink when I graduated from eighth grade. My father gave me a cigarette and a drink. It was kind of like a Portuguese bar mitzvah. We went from having very rigid rules until we got to high school, and then, all of a sudden, we were kind of cut loose. We could do whatever we wanted. Once I started drinking, I could not stop. I just drank to oblivion, just like with food.

It was a fad in our neighborhood to steal. We stole from the local stores, and I never did get caught. But I remember feeling guilty about it. The first time I stole something, I was probably around seven or eight. It was from a drugstore in our neighborhood. I felt so bad about it that I went home and wouldn't let myself eat dinner. We also used to terrorize our neighborhood. We'd wait until everybody was asleep at night, and we would go around throwing garbage cans down the hill. We'd make noise with them clanking and racing, and would do other crazy stuff. We fought a lot. One of the ways to get respect was to be tough and bad. That was the sort of James Dean kind of ideal.

I was shy with girls in high school and didn't date much. But I fell in love my senior year with a girl who was as crazy as I was. The relationship was about drinking, arguing, fighting, and also around sex. I was hopelessly in love, and when we split up, I just could not get over it. I just kept hanging around, and we dated on and off. At that point in my life, once I was attached to something, I was not willing to let go.

The fat got in the way of relationships for a while after that. I felt very self-conscious without a T-shirt on because I had the rolls and the breasts and stuff. On the one hand, I was very embarrassed by my body, and on the other hand, I had loads of testosterone and normal male urges.

By the time my first big relationship ended, I just did not know what to do next. I was so self-conscious and wounded. It was awhile before I had another girlfriend. When I was about twenty-one, I met Sandy who was five years younger than I was. Her mother didn't like me, and of course, that made me more determined to see this girl. I liked her, and I loved her in my own bizarre way, as much as a compulsive overeating, alcoholic can love anybody when they're in their disease. We got married, simply because I had no self-esteem.

At that time, I was working on a furniture and upholstery cleaning truck and going to college part-time. My father was the first member of his family to get a college education, and because he was Irish, he valued his education. In a way, I was trying to prove myself to him by going to college and getting good grades. But sometimes the drinking and partying got in the way, so I went in and out of school.

My marriage to Sandy lasted about three years. Her sexual boundaries were nonexistent. She slept with anybody she wanted to. And I took it really personally. I was the fat kid who was drinking and had no self-esteem. Finally, I couldn't take it anymore. One night when she didn't come home, I wouldn't let her back in the house. We wound up going back and forth, but nothing changed. I tried to talk to her about her infidelity, but I knew she lied to me. Short of hiring a detective, there was nothing I could do about it. She was going to do what she was going to do, and I could not live with that. It had already made me crazy.

By the time we got divorced I had dropped out of college and was working as a truck driver. Since I belonged to a really powerful union, as long as I did my job there was nothing anyone could do to me. I could wear my hair as long as I wanted, I could dress funny, act weird, anything I wanted to. I was drinking like a fish and was just out of control. I lost weight during this period because of depression and because of the drinking. I wasn't eating a lot, and I got down to a pretty normal size.

A few years later I got married again, even though I knew at the time it was a bad idea. Again, because my self-esteem was so low, I figured if someone would have me, then I will marry her. Sarah and I fought all the time, very ugly fighting. It was a vicious, vicious marriage. I used to tell people that I spent ten years in a two-year marriage.

Two days after we got married, I was in a really bad accident on my motorcycle. A woman made an illegal turn and plowed her car into me. When I got to the hospital, I was on life support and was pretty close to dying. The femoral artery in one of my legs was severed. I had about twelve surgeries during that first year to repair all the injuries. But they couldn't save my leg, and eventually they had to amputate it.

When I was in the hospital, I naturally spent a lot of time wondering whether I was going to live or die. I decided I wanted a child, someone to carry on the family name. Scott was born a year after the accident. I couldn't go back to work, and was on disability, so I became a house-husband which actually wasn't that bad. But I was very depressed about my physical condition and in a terrible marriage, so I started overeating again on a daily basis. I would eat five Kit Kat candy bars for just a snack. I would go to the market and pick up seven hot dogs, give my son one, and I would eat the rest.

I got suicidal after the amputation, and it was serious. I put a large caliber handgun in my mouth with six rounds in it, which was insane because it only takes one round and that quick squeeze. But I just had had enough. Then I took the gun out of my mouth and started to cry and to grieve. My mother died during this time too. She had been in the hospital for emphysema. It's hard to describe how awful I felt.

At this point, I got into therapy for the first time. I was in therapy for three or four years, and it was helpful up to a certain extent. But often, I would leave the therapist's office and pick up five or six donuts to eat on the way home, and then pick up a bottle of wine to have with dinner. You cannot do therapy and addiction at the same time. So, I just kind of ran out of gas in therapy, and there was nothing left to do there.

My second destructive marriage had ended, and I went back to school to get a bachelor's and master's degree in psychology. I was still out of control with my eating, but my drinking was mostly limited to weekends. After I got my degrees, I went to work for a social service agency. My weight had ballooned up again to between 320–350 pounds. A man I worked with mentioned that there was a really good program called Overeaters Anonymous that I might want to check out. I was tired of feeling so isolated and depressed about my eating, so I decided to try it. After the first meeting, I was so impressed by the program and the people in it. I remember seeing these people had lost weight, and they seemed happy and were having a good time. And I went to my second meeting and realized this was it.

I got a sponsor who had lost 110 pounds, and that was certainly an attraction for me. About three months later, I got a step sponsor and started working the steps. I started losing weight like you wouldn't believe. It was about fifteen pounds a month. I started at around 320 pounds and got down to 163 in eleven months. I was praying and meditating, even though I was an atheist. It seemed like as long as I kept going to those meetings, and kept working those steps, and talking in meetings, and connecting with people, I knew I was safe and that this would work.

It was abnormal for me to be connected to a group of people and depending on them, and it was like a miracle this gift that I was given. I trusted these people, some of them, not all of them, and I knew they had what I wanted. I just had to be willing to do the work, take the emotional inventories, and not do the addiction in between.

While I worked through the steps, I got to take inventory of the people I resented and was angry toward. I wrote thirteen angry pages about my father, and the theme of humiliation ran all through it. I went deeper and deeper into my childhood, and the family alcoholism and abuse. I was able also to look at my middle brother's sadism and sexual advances toward me. I never went along with him, but still, it was disturbing.

After my second OA meeting, I have been abstinent to this day. The way I've been abstinent has changed, but I have never gained the weight back. I am probably around 175 pounds now. Back then, being abstinent meant eating four ounces of protein three times a day, and fruit and vegetables, and that was it. Flour and grains were considered taboo. I have gradually added stuff back, like flour and grains. I still weigh and measure breakfast today and I eyeball my other meals, but I weighed and measured for the first seven years I was in the program.

I quit drinking when I started OA. It was not good for you, and it was also additional calories. I started swimming for exercise and became a pretty good distance swimmer, and even competed in some masters swim competitions. I married a third time, and it was a much healthier relationship than the others.

Now I would say my self-esteem is pretty good. I never did like the term "self-love," and thought I would settle with liking myself seventy-five percent of the time. I probably feel good about myself about 90 percent of the time now. I don't have a problem with anger anymore, although if someone corners me and threatens me, it is still there. I think I am softer now, more loving, and more supportive of the people I care about. I'm also more direct if I am upset about something, or don't agree with something. I am more willing to stand up for myself.

I love both my parents now, even though they are dead. I spent a lot of time in the past feeling like a victim and hating both of them. Now I admire them both for their good qualities. My mom was a piece of work, but she taught me a lot, especially the love of poetry and music and reading.

I like my job as an administrator for a social service agency. I get to help people with their problems and supervise about fifteen employees.

My relationships with others, including my wife, are much more balanced and sane now.

My spiritual life has changed too. I don't understand the concept of God and how miracles supposedly happen. But I do think, now, that God exists. It's hard to understand God on an intellectual basis; I think it can only be understood in your heart, and then only partially. All I know is that at this point in my life, I feel much more at peace, and it's a great feeling.

6

EMILY

Emily is 28, married, and has two children. She was anorexic from the age of thirteen until her freshman year of college.

My memories of my early childhood are mostly happy ones. Our family was really close, and we were always doing family things. My dad had his own insurance business, and my mom was a stay-at-home mom. She volunteered outside the home, and did watercolor painting and other art in her spare time. I had a sister two years older than me, and four younger brothers and sisters.

I think one important issue for me was the need to stand out and be different because I was in a family of six kids. I especially tried to be different from my older sister, one way or the other. Since I felt she was smarter than me in school, I had to find other ways to excel.

As a young child I was always thought of as "the pretty one" compared to her. I had lighter hair and a fairer complexion than Julie. My dad would tell me nice things that people said when he showed them our photo, such as "Oh, wow, look at that pretty blonde girl." I cared more about my appearance than Julie cared about hers. She was very confident and didn't feel she had to prove anything to anyone else, whereas I was always trying to look good for others and trying to impress them.

I remember always wanting my mom's attention, but she was constantly busy because she had six kids, so I never seemed to get one-on-one attention. When I'd ask her to do something with me, she'd say she didn't have time, that she had to fix dinner, or do laundry, or take care of one of the other kids.

My mom had a hard time expressing her feelings, whether it was a hug or verbally saying, "I love you." I don't think her parents were very affectionate, so feelings are very hard for her. Even now, if I talk to her on the phone and say, "I love you," she will not say it back, though I know she loves me. Unlike my mom, my dad is a very loving, touchy person. He's very relaxed and easy to be with. I felt like I got a lot of attention from him.

Another way I managed to stand out in my family was through sports. I was very confident about my athletic abilities. When we were in elementary school, my mom put Julie and me on a swim team, and in ballet and track. Julie was a much better dancer, and it turned out that I was much better in sports. So I played soccer, and I swam, and I ran.

I was really good at running, and I did that for a long time. It was something I shared with my dad because he came to all my track meets and cheered for me. I loved the time I had with him, and I thought I was more important than Julie to him because I did sports. So, naturally this made me feel quite special.

Eventually, when I was in eighth grade, the competition got too much for me. I was such a perfectionist; I won every race and was so good at track, until one day another girl on my team beat me. I just couldn't handle it, that someone could beat me. At that point, I decided to find something to be good at that no one else could do. I had such a need to stand out and be an individual. So I started eating less and focusing on that. I think I purposely threw myself out of the competition because I couldn't handle it anymore.

Eating had always been a focal point in our house. My mom was basically a weird eater. She would not sit down with us when we had dinner and eat; she would have just a tiny bit and say she was not hungry. Then we would see her afterward, staying in the kitchen and eating. I think that this was huge for me. To stand out and be validated by my mom, I felt like you could not eat. I remember, as a young child, if you went into the kitchen to get a cookie, she would always be like, "Do not eat any more cookies, what are you doing?" She very much controlled what we ate.

My sister, Julie, was always getting put down for what she ate. We would be on vacation and my mom would tell her, "Oh, if you keep eating like that, you won't be able to fit in your clothes when you get home." I remember thinking I wanted my mom to think I was better than Julie, so I thought I would never eat that way. My mom did not want fat kids; she cared a lot about the way her kids looked. She cared how we appeared to others, and that we appear as a very put-together, happy, perfect family.

My eating patterns started to change in the spring of eighth grade. I would come home from school, eat just a little, and then go to both swimming and track. One night after these two workouts, my family went out to eat. I ordered a caramel sundae, as always, because that was my favorite thing. My mom told me I really should order something healthy because I had been exercising. I think now she just meant I should get a meal, but then I took it to mean I was bad, that something was wrong with me because I wanted ice cream. I remember feeling very nervous and anxious, and telling the waitress to change my order to a sandwich instead. I was so black or white in my thinking. I thought to myself, "Ice cream is bad, so I can never eat ice cream again." When everyone else got ice cream that night, I felt like I was a better person because I only had a sandwich.

I was already skinny enough. I never thought I was fat. I liked having so much control, and thinking I was a stronger person than everyone else. I just started exercising more and more, and eating less and less. I started stepping on the scale a lot, and then thinking I really could lose more weight because I am so good at this.

I started getting a lot of attention. The track coach said something to my mom because I was becoming a slower runner, and he pulled me aside one day and talked to me about what I should be eating. I acted like I didn't like the extra attention, but I must have actually liked it.

My mom took me to see a dietitian who told me what foods to eat for extra energy, and that it was okay to have a cookie sometimes. But I labeled sweets as terrible foods that I would never eat. I thought to myself that I will make my own decisions, and no one can control what I eat. Not eating was my sole way of rebelling. I was such a perfect child in almost every other way.

Eventually, I got weaker and weaker. My coaches told my mom I was too great a liability for them, and that I would have to leave the track and swim teams. As I got kicked out of things, I got more and more angry. I thought, "Well, you guys can try and kick me out of everything, but you can't control anything I do." And I kept getting skinnier and skinnier.

That summer, when I was thirteen, I became an exercise fanatic. In the morning, I ate a tiny amount of cereal or else some peaches with a little milk. Then I left the house and walked all over. I couldn't run because the ligaments in my leg felt too weird, but I walked for hours and hours. I chewed on a lot of gum and drank diet cokes. I made sure I was not home for dinnertime, and I would come in late. My mother saved me dinner, but I waited until she wasn't paying attention and gave most of it to one of my brothers to eat, or threw it away. I would just have a bunch of vegetables. Then I waited until everyone went to bed to sneak into the kitchen and eat. I didn't want anyone to see me eat because I thought it was a bad thing. I didn't even realize at the time that I was copying some of my mother's eating behavior.

I never ate as little as other girls with anorexia I've read about. I ate only small amounts, no fat, and definitely less than 1,000 calories a day, but I didn't restrict myself to one piece of bread or a couple of grapes. I exercised three or more hours a day. Sometimes, if I felt mad, I'd go into my room to do jumping jacks. I never did laxatives because I thought that was weak, and I had to be strong. My best friend was bulimic. She would eat a whole loaf of bread and then throw it up. I tried purging a few times, but I never did it. I never ate too much where I needed to purge. I just had this ultimate control over what I put in my mouth.

Finally, during my freshman year of high school, my mom said she'd had enough of watching me waste away and insisted I go for counseling. I think it was very hard for her to admit I needed counseling and that she couldn't take care of my problems herself. The first counselor I saw had me sit on one side of a mirror with her, and my parents or other people sat on the other side and watched. That was humiliating and didn't work. Then my mom found someone else who I liked, though I was determined not to let anyone change me.

My counselor insisted that I have regular doctors' appointments to be weighed and examined. I was very conniving. I knew if my weight was too low, I would be put in the hospital. The only time I allowed myself to eat sweets and binge was the night before an appointment. I would stuff myself with animal crackers, vanilla wafers, and other snacks. At the doctor's office, I told my mother I did not want her in the room with me, and then I would go in the bathroom and drink so much water I thought I would die. I would wear these big heavy clothes, stuff jewelry in my pockets, and convince the nurse to weigh me with my clothes on.

This worked for a while, but I was still over-exercising. I was always out walking at every opportunity, as fast as I could. Sometimes guys would scream out of their cars, "You're so disgusting, you're so skinny," things like that, and it would totally hurt my feelings. I felt like no one could relate to me. I am very much a "people person," but the worse I got, the more depressed I got. My two closest friends pulled out of my life because they couldn't handle it. Their parents told them to stay away from me. No one wanted to do things with me, no guys wanted to ask me out, I didn't go to any school dances. I remember thinking how everyone hated me.

My mom was very worried and very angry. I knew she loved me, but sometimes she was so mad at me it felt like she hated me. She would drive me to the doctor for my weigh-in, and she wouldn't talk to me at all. At home, she sometimes gave me the silent treatment for twenty-four hours at a time. I realize now how much I hurt her at the time, but I didn't see that then. She sometimes told me, "You're going to die," and I remember thinking, "Good, I would like to die." I basically thought if I died it would be better for everyone, but I never thought of actually killing myself.

I had to see a nutritionist several times, but she couldn't help me. She would give me these meal plans, and it just seemed like such an abundance of food to me. I knew I was supposed to eat, but I could not do it on my own. It was too hard.

Eventually, I couldn't keep my weight up, even with my deceptions, and I had to go into the hospital. I am 5'7" tall, and I weighed 85 pounds when I was first hospitalized. It was Thanksgiving of my junior year. In the hospital they had me on 2500 calories a day, and I had to gain one-half pound a day in order to watch TV or have visitors. Even though I drank a ton of water first, I had to be weighed in a hospital gown, and I never gained the half-pound a day very easily. I don't remember this as much as my family does, but that Thanksgiving Day they all came to visit me, and I could not see them. My mom cried, and they were all very upset.

In the hospital, I would take the food they gave me and hide it whenever I could. One time, the doctor came in and found my butter stashed somewhere. I was very embarrassed. I often closed my drapes and exercised in my room. They kind of stuck me in my room and said to eat, but it was very hard for me because I could not talk to anyone about it. I just got angry or upset, and developed weird habits. It didn't help me develop good eating habits at all. They didn't offer any treatment. I would finally get released, then lose the weight, and have to go back in again. That happened two or three times.

I was never content with the way I looked, but I wasn't the type to look in the mirror and think I was obese. I did think I looked disgusting and ugly, and that I was hopeless. That was it more than anything.

Sometimes I thought I looked bigger, and that was scary, but mainly my obsession was driven by the need for power and control.

In my junior year, I started getting progressively worse. Finally, one day as we were driving to the doctor's for a weigh-in, I told my mom that I was down to 68 pounds. I remember thinking that I could not do this anymore. I could not drink all the water anymore. The last time I'd been weighed in, I felt so sick from all the water when I left the doctor's office that I threw up before I got to the car. I felt so dizzy, and I thought how I was just killing myself. I guess, at that point, I wasn't ready to kill myself and was ready for help. The doctor's office thought I weighed 85 pounds because of all my tricks, but I let them weigh me in a hospital gown. They were so upset that I had done all this and they hadn't known, and that I was so much sicker than they thought.

My counselor recommended that my family send me to a local hospital's eating disorders treatment program, and that's what they did. It was a huge benefit being there all day, every day. It was a necessity for me to be out of school, and out of normal life, and to focus on my problem that needed to be fixed. I made a few friends in the program who were dealing with the same things, people who were a lot like me.

I felt a lot of pressure at school because I felt like I did not fit in. In this program, I felt like I was okay because I did not have to try to fit in. I did not have to try to be something I was not. I did not have to try to talk to people if I didn't want to. There were a lot of things I did not have to do. I really enjoyed not having to please anyone or having to smile for anyone if I did not want to smile. I think in some respects I would have liked to be a quiet person, but I always felt like I was supposed to be outgoing and talkative and happy. I did not fit in because I made myself not fit in, but I didn't realize that at the time. So I just thought, "No one likes me, I am just weird, and I just don't fit in anywhere." I hated going to school, and getting me out of there, out of my environment, helped me get rid of some of my depression. I felt like I was validated here, that these people liked me.

It helped that I was forced to eat, but not by myself, like in the hospital. We all ate together. There were very normal girls there who were just like me, and they were struggling to eat, just like me. I felt we were all in this together. There was also one girl I would watch who was much older than me, in her thirties, and I thought she was very weird. I thought how I could become like this girl, and how I didn't want to go on living my life like this.

They monitored us while we ate, and I remember thinking how this wasn't that hard. I didn't have to decide what to eat, the food was good, and we had to eat it. Afterward, instead of being alone and feeling antsy and full and fat, we sat together in a group and talked about how we felt, or just listened to each other. It forced me to see that I could eat a whole meal, feel full, and still be alive and okay. I was not gaining ten pounds a day. They weighed us once a week and I never looked at the scale; I turned my back so I couldn't see. I felt safe. They told me what I was gaining each day, usually about one-half a pound a day. I think it kind of jump-started me, and got me to gain that initial weight.

The program offered a lot of group counseling which helped, but I didn't like the classes where we had to act things out, or do art and draw our feelings. I was just not into that. I saw a psychiatrist there because everyone did, and he recommended that I go on Prozac. But my mom said absolutely not. I don't know why she felt so strongly, but it helped me to have people realize I was depressed.

I stayed in this program for a month. It was terrifying to face going back to school. I was so afraid of what people would say, and how I would feel about it. Most people just said I looked really good, and I know, the first day back, I took it as people think I am fat now. But my counseling sessions helped me deal with my feelings and my insecurities about my appearance, and with all my other issues too. Finally, I just accepted that I was okay. I think, before that, I didn't want to look good because I didn't want to have to live up to the pressure of having to look good. I didn't want to have to be pretty and cute; I just wanted to be left alone to be my own self.

After that, I was able to maintain a stable weight of about 95 pounds until I left home to go to college in another state. It was so liberating at college to be able to start all over. I was completely removed from my environment, and I made all new friends. No one knew anything at all about my eating disorder. No one was telling me, "You're looking so good" or "You're looking so healthy." I had fun and completely forgot I had this disorder.

I don't know if it was reverse psychology or what, but my mom told me several times that if I couldn't keep my weight up, they would have to bring me home. And I remember thinking, there was no way they were going to make me come home.

My roommate became my best friend, and she was so good for me. She was very carefree, and she showed me the fun of hanging out, and eating, and staying up late at night, instead of getting up every day and exercising. I was ready to forget my old unhealthy sick self, and have fun, and be liked by guys. I gradually let go of all the control I had tried to have. It wasn't always easy for me, though. I still wasn't totally relaxed when I ate. I would force myself to eat what everyone else ate because I wanted to fit in. Sometimes, after we ate a lot of junk food, I felt antsy and went out running, even if it was at night and wintertime. I felt a little bit lost for a while, but I just let it happen. I would have a night like that, but then I would go back and be normal.

I felt so popular during college. I was very social and went out almost every night. People liked me and approved of me, and guys thought I looked good. I loved my classes, and studied a lot, so that part went well too. I didn't have a scale, and I don't remember thinking about my weight much at all. I knew I was gaining weight because my clothes weren't fitting, but that was okay, and my roommate was so positive. She said, "Let's take a picture of you in all your clothes, so your mom will buy you more clothes when you go home."

My first visit home, I remember being a little nervous about whether people would think I was too big. By then I weighed 120 pounds. But the son of one of my mom's friends saw me and told his mom how gorgeous I looked. That was all I needed to hear, and then it was fine.

There were a few difficult periods for me during the next years. Early in my junior year, I roomed with a girl who was bulimic, though I didn't know this at the time. We were really good friends and would stay up late, eating a lot, and studying. I got chunkier than I had ever been. I remember going home, and my mom telling me it was not a good weight for me, that I had to find a weight that was right for me. It was really hard for me to hear that. I returned to school and became more obsessive about my food and exercise.

I went running every single day, even if it was pitch black outside, or pouring down rain. I still ate meals, but not as much, though I would eat frozen yogurt like it was going out of style. I did get the weight off, but I never let it get super low. Eventually, I stabilized and felt okay again.

I met my husband when we were both students. He is a very laid-back person who is so good for me. He is not hard on me about anything. He's changed my confidence level tremendously because I feel so unconditionally loved. He's always telling me that I look good, that I'm good at doing things, and that he appreciates me. We got married right after my graduation. We stayed in the same college community while he finished his graduate work, and I got a job in a local florist shop.

Right after we were married, I had another slight relapse. I joined a gym and went there early in the mornings before work. I made a group of friends there who were all early morning exercisers like me. Somehow, it got really competitive with us to see who was coming in at 5 A.M., and how long each of us was exercising. One girl was getting skinnier and skinnier, and wasn't eating much, and we both got kind of competitive with each other. If my alarm went off late and Amanda beat me to the gym, I thought I was a bad person. Every morning I would be there by 5 A.M. and exercise until 8 A.M., every single day.

I didn't realize how thin I was getting until people started making comments. One day at work, I was eating lunch at my desk and someone came in with a delivery and said, "Oh, you actually eat." My husband was really worried and thought maybe he had done something that made me lose weight. Finally, when I was visiting my family during Christmas, my mom warned me that I might have to go back into the hospital if I wasn't careful. I remember thinking, "I will not!" I knew I looked bad; at that point I was down to 100 pounds. I didn't want people to think of me like the way I used to be because I didn't feel I was like that anymore. And I wanted to be able to get pregnant eventually, but at this weight I wasn't even getting my period.

Another reason I was determined to get healthy again was that one of my younger sisters started showing signs of an eating disorder. That really threw me over the edge. I felt like I was a terrible example to her. She confided in me, and we talked on the phone a lot. Fortunately, she never got to the point that I did, but I think if I hadn't had a problem, and my mom wasn't the way she was, maybe my sister wouldn't have struggled with an eating disorder at all.

I gradually regained the weight I had lost and stopped exercising so compulsively. But it took me almost two years to get pregnant when we decided to start a family. The main side effects from my anorexia were irregular periods and infertility. I've also had some small bone fractures, like a hairline fracture in my foot when I was working out three hours a day. I thought maybe my bones were brittle from the anorexia, but I haven't had any other problems since I've had children. Of course, now I'm taking good care of myself and eating well.

I think I have come so far, but I also think because of who I am that I may never lose the pressure to watch what I eat. I probably think more about my weight and appearance than a person who hasn't been through what I have. But it's not really an obsession anymore. When I've been pregnant, I've made sure I am very healthy, and I gain the twenty-five to thirty-five pounds that are recommended. Afterward, though, I'm not completely satisfied until I've taken off the weight. I do it gradually, and try not to obsess about it too much, since it does take time to get it off in a healthy way.

I still exercise at a gym every morning before my husband goes to work. But I no longer get up quite as early, and one hour is enough of a workout for me. Even when I have more time to exercise, I don't have the drive in me anymore. I have so many other things going on in my life now. I love everything about being a mother. My joy lies in being a wife and mother. I love having the companionship of my husband and not being in any type of competition. He values me, and I know I am so important to him and my kids. I have lots of friends, but my life is more with my family.

I'm more relaxed now than I have ever been. I've been able to let go of some of my perfectionism. If the house isn't clean or decorated perfectly, it's okay. Feeling that I am an individual, and that I am important, makes me much happier than having to prove myself to other people.

Now, I am trying not to repeat past mistakes. My husband and I have talked about ground rules for our kids, especially our two-year old daughter. We don't talk much about food or weight or appearance. I try to be conscious of what I say and do with my life because my little girl watches everything I do. The world already focuses enough on bodies and images, and I think it is even harder if it comes from your home too. Critical parents create children with all sorts of problems. I think children need a lot of unconditional love, and to feel valued for all their special qualities.

7

CHRISTINA

Christina is a 42-year-old, married book editor who had problems with compulsive overeating for eighteen years. She has been recovered for more than six years.

Looking back, my eating disorder really started when I was in junior high school. I would wake up and have just a glass of orange juice for breakfast and a fudgesicle for lunch. Then I would basically not eat until I came home from school, and then I would eat anything I wanted. This would include a great amount of sugar and caffeine, things like a grilled cheese sandwich, lots of potato chips, two or three candy bars, and two or three cokes. The only time I would have a balanced meal was at dinner when my family ate together, though that was only about half the week. There were no rules for food in my home, so I wound up practically fasting for half the day and then gorging the other half. We always had a huge amount of sweets and snack foods around.

Probably because I was a dancer and pretty skinny, I was able to eat a lot of food and not gain weight. The way I ate then didn't feel neurotic to me. I didn't think much about it. I had other problems to think about instead.

Growing up, I remember always having the feeling of being an outsider in my own family. My two older brothers could do no wrong. They were smart and athletic, and were always joking around with my mom. Compared to them, I felt too dumb, too young, too boring, or too much trouble. They both treated me in a disdainful way, always being impatient with me and calling me stupid.

My mom was busy, busy, busy, so I have the experience of her carting me places in the car, but I don't remember ever sitting down and having an actual conversation with her. We had a very superficial relationship. She did not have a sense of who I was and didn't bother to try to find out. She wanted things easy and hopeful and nice, and if I talked for more than a few sentences, she would get impatient. So what was missing for me was patience and a depth of understanding.

Then there was my father...almost the opposite of my mother. He was a college history professor and a very serious person. It would have been nice to have had some ease and superficiality with my dad instead of worry, criticism, and heavy conversations. He was the disciplinarian, while my mom attempted to be the peacemaker. Being angry and arguing or shouting weren't stood for, so if any of us would talk back, pretty soon Dad's voice would raise and say, "We are not going to stand for this. I am going to wash your mouth out with soap." He would physically drag me to the bathroom and shove soap in my mouth. I would have a moment of being scared when I saw him coming after me, and then I would numb out. And then I would be sort of seething. In my room, I never had tantrums or got out the anger; it just got buried.

When my father criticized me about something, I would take it to heart and would assume he was right all the time. It was important to him that I follow certain rules of behavior in the world and fit in. He was very strict. If I didn't say hello quickly enough to an adult who stopped by the house, he would reprimand me. If I had a different opinion about our church or a person we both knew, he would make me feel wrong and bad. His love felt very conditional, like he would withdraw it if I didn't act in a certain way.

The memories I had when I was a kid were so much about trying to fit in, trying hard to be the kind of kid I suspected that my parents wanted, or that my brothers wanted.

I remember always feeling so inadequate. At dinner, my brothers were on one side of the table, next to each other, and I was on the other side. They would laugh and joke with each other, and with my mom, and I always felt like I didn't belong.

I think I put on a pretty good face. No one thought I was unhappy; instead people considered me cute and playful. We had a good life. We had what we needed and weren't struggling for money. But as I look back, my childhood wasn't a normal one because I went around with an internal kind of gloom, no matter how successful I was on the outside.

Dancing became an outlet for me. When I was four or five, my mother put me into a creative dance class, and that was a place where I could shine. From age seven until I left for college, I took ballet in a neighborhood dance studio. There were people with all types of body shapes, and my body image was pretty darn good. Even when my body developed and I wasn't as skinny, it was okay with me.

In high school, I was editor of the yearbook, in the gymnastics team, and held various offices in student government. I had friends in different groups in school—popular, and not so popular—so I was able to fit in, socially, pretty easily. But I remember being jealous of friends a lot, especially if they had close, happy families, and always feeling like there was something wrong with me.

During this time, I had some experiences that my parents never discovered. I had sex with my first serious boyfriend when I was fifteen. I didn't feel guilty at all, but I was worried about getting pregnant. I experimented with smoking cigarettes when I was thirteen, and smoked a half a pack a day for a few years. I tried marijuana when I was fourteen, and then speed, but really didn't use drugs very much at all. I shoplifted a little, just to see what I could get away with.

Both my brothers went to Ivy League schools, so naturally I was expected to do the same. I was torn between wanting to audition with a ballet company in Ohio, where we lived, and go to college at night, and wanting to follow in my brothers' footsteps. And, of course, my parents had strong opinions about which choice I should make. So I never knew if I went to Princeton to please myself, or just to please others. All I know is that I became depressed pretty quickly. I probably had the makings of depression before I even got there.

It was hard to be around all these really smart people, and to see them genuinely happy to be there, with goals and purpose, and not confused about their lives like I was. I started on birth control pills soon after I got to college. I would not be surprised if the pill, with all the hormonal changes, contributed to my depression. It certainly contributed to a huge weight gain, especially in my breasts. I went from a size C to a DD cup, which totally changed my self-image around being a dancer type. Suddenly I was just this curvy woman; I didn't like that. I remember my sophomore year having a professor who seemed to have a crush on me. He came to see me perform, and I was wearing a leotard. It made me really uncomfortable to start being looked at, and feel objectified by men, because of my breasts.

Pretty soon, I started eating lots and lots of sugar—cookies while I was studying and marshmallow fluff—and eating second dinners later in the evening. I wound up gaining twenty pounds in about one month. At some point, I tried to throw up, and I couldn't. I knew I wasn't going to let myself gain more weight, especially since I was determined to continue dance classes and performing while at Princeton, so I started controlling my weight by skipping meals. I was either bingeing or dieting, and was eating most of my calories in bad food.

I knew I had a problem, and I went to seek help. I did not have any judgment about going to see a therapist. I only had a couple of sessions, though, because the person I picked could not quite fully understand or hear me; she just could not break through that shield surrounding me.

I was close to people in college, but never really found soul mates there. This contributed to my sense of loneliness, and it probably started my experience of going to men; if I could not have really good friendships, at least I could have a boyfriend. I would have one guy who was my best friend and lover, and when we broke up, I would have another best friend and lover as soon as possible. I continued like this through my twenties, not having any close friends other than boyfriends.

After college, I lived in Philadelphia for a while and then moved to California to live with some friends I knew from college. I bounced back and forth between jobs, trying to decide whether to use my intellect or my artistic self. I still danced after work, in dance studios and in local dance productions, so I kind of got away with having an eating disorder. I was eating lots of sugar, and there were often times when a meal would consist of a piece of fruit and three large chocolate chip cookies. I would eat a pound bag of M&M's in one sitting and just eat less the next day. It was sort of controlled bingeing at that point and was not a really big deal yet. What was more of a big deal was the depression.

My sexuality started getting out of hand. I just did not feel good about myself, and one way to feel good was to feel wanted. I lost count of how many lovers I had. Often, I was drunk or stoned or on cocaine when I was having sex. I would always binge afterwards. I still felt somewhat in control of my eating; I would just binge, feel sick, and diet the next day.

I pretty much fell apart when I was twenty-six, and the publishing company I worked for at the time transferred me to Phoenix. I didn't know anyone there, and I got more and more depressed. I quit my job because I was not feeling right. I started applying to go back to school, thinking maybe I would get a Ph.D. in English. I had this sort of grandiose view of what I could do, but I could not follow through. During this time, I got a job working for minimum wage packing boxes with materials, and I could not keep that job either.

There was a numbness to this whole depression time, and a numbness about reality and denial that I needed to live with. I could not believe that here I was, twenty-six, a Princeton graduate, so skilled, so talented, and so dysfunctional. I could not really face that I lived with a cloud over me. Part of the cloud was eating poorly too, and it soothed me. One of my favorite soothing foods was raw cookie batter, or raw brownie batter. They were soft and gooey, and helped me feel okay and numb.

My eating got out of control. I would wake up and eat raw brownie batter for breakfast. I would basically go through days of eating nothing but sugar. I couldn't vomit, but I would be sick to my stomach. After two or three days of eating like this, I would feel so sick that I didn't want to eat. So I wouldn't eat for a day or two, and then the whole cycle would start up again. I was just so compulsively eating chocolate and sugar that I couldn't stop. By this time I was about thirty pounds heavier than I wanted to be, and that was always on my mind.

Finally, I went to a therapist who recommended that I get on medication. A psychiatrist prescribed an anti-psychotic drug for me that I tried for a few months. I had a lot of side effects, and it didn't help my depression at all. When I went back to ask for a different medication, the psychiatrist just defended his decision and refused to prescribe something else. So I went off this drug cold turkey, and that was basically the bottom. Going cold turkey off this drug had me suicidal. I played with razor blades one morning, but I knew I did not have it in me to really do it. I thought about standing in front of trucks on the highway. I mean I really wanted it over; I just felt so hopeless.

A few of my new friends saw the struggles I was going through, but felt powerless to help. Most people, though, didn't take my problems seriously when I talked about them because I was able to present a good front. I wanted to get someone to put me into a hospital, but I sounded too good. It felt like I was playing out this thing from childhood again, of nobody really seeing me.

I moved back to California, where it felt more familiar and I had a little more support. I found a psychiatrist who put me on an appropriate antidepressant, and the suicidal tendency diminished into almost nothing. When I was suicidal, I was acting very inappropriate sexually—propositioning a couple of married friends, for example—but that behavior went away as soon as I was on antidepressants. That tells me now, in hindsight, that my biochemistry was being altered because of how much sugar I was eating.

Soon, I got a job working in a small bookstore. One of my coworkers was in AA and invited me to go with her to a meeting. I thought I'd go to just kind of support her and see what she was going through. Well, I wound up crying through the whole meeting. They were telling my story. For me it had nothing to do with alcohol; it had to do with sugar or chocolate or eating. For the first time in twenty-seven years, I saw other people who were dealing with this. I could talk honestly and openly, and not have someone say, "You look fine to me."

After that, I attended Overeaters Anonymous meetings for about five years. OA was my main way of finding myself again. It offered me a safe haven in which to explore the multi-faceted relationship I had with food. Food had become my best friend and my worst enemy, my comfort and my self-destruction. It took time for me to be ready to change. The first few months I went to meetings, I was bingeing severely, and still in a cycle of bingeing and dieting, bingeing and dieting. At two in the morning, I would put a coat over my pajamas, and go to Safeway to buy more cookies and candy. I would eat until I was just sick, and then I could barely fall asleep because my stomach hurt so much.

I had mentors in OA who helped teach me how to eat. With their help, I figured out how to eat three balanced meals and two snacks a day, and it felt opulent. I did not feel like I was dieting at all, but I also didn't gain any weight. I started learning that recovery from compulsive overeating was not going to be a quick fix. I remember saying at an OA meeting one evening that the day I finally stopped impatiently measuring the time I was taking to lose those extra thirty pounds was, ironically, the day I started to lose weight.

I still saw a therapist because I knew I still needed to do the inner work, but I changed therapists several times before I found the one who helped me the most. I joined a support group, based on Geneen Roth's work, where I learned to explore new ways of self-acceptance. I went to a personal growth workshop where I listed one of my goals as making peace with my relationship to food. Between part one and part two of this workshop, I woke up one day and decided I would choose, one day at a time, not to eat chocolate. It seemed that chocolate was always the starting point for my worst binges.

Eventually, I stopped going to OA because I had already gotten much of what I needed out of it. I didn't want to stick with the whole 12-step thing and being told I was powerless. I went from thinking my therapist was my higher power, to maybe God could be my higher power, to the idea that I could incorporate my own inner knowledge and inner power to guide me to the right choices. As soon as I began to depend more on myself, I lost what I called the black hole in my stomach, and I stopped bingeing.

Other experiences helped along the way. One summer I volunteered to lead backpacking trips in the mountains. Mastering a new skill, and having strength and power in a functional way that was of service, made a huge difference that summer. One inheritance from my father, which I greatly appreciate, is his love of nature. I started making it a priority to go into nature and be with myself, whether it was to sit on a rock and cry, or to hug a tree. Both in times of pain and joy, I wanted to find a sense through nature of what God might be for me.

My work in therapy was mostly about me learning how to have a healthy relationship with another person, and also to come to terms with my past. I began to realize that my parents' and brothers' inadequacies were more to do with them than with me. I still felt hurt and angry, at times, at the way they treated me (and continued to treat me), but I also started trying to look at what was good in these relationships. I learned ways to communicate my feelings to them when I didn't feel good about what they did or said. And I found people, friends, and other members of support groups I joined, who were able to give me the emotional backing I needed. As a result, I gradually became less critical and rejecting of myself. If I had a small binge, or procrastinated, or didn't exercise after I thought I was going to, I was able to be more forgiving and compassionate with myself.

As I felt stronger, the nature of my relationship with men began to change. Since high school, I had not been able to have guys as friends. The attitude I carried around, that they either wanted to criticize me or sleep with me, kept me from getting close to them. I was finally able to develop some healthy platonic relationships with guys. And when I did see someone in a dating sense, if it was clear we weren't compatible, we could finish off very easily, and often remain on friendly terms. I made more positive choices, and learned more about myself, as I went along.

Eventually, I met my husband, Dave, who is a great partner for me. We met four years ago through some mutual friends. He had been married briefly once before, ten years earlier. Dave had gone through some counseling during the years, and was pretty aware of his own "stuff." We have many similar values and interests, and have a really healthy relationship.

One difficult thing I've had to accept is that, for now, I still need to be on an antidepressant. For a few years I did fine without medication, but about seven years ago I got really depressed again. I was still functional, but I became more self-critical to the point where I didn't see any hope. I had a very short fuse and got hopeless pretty quickly. I decided it wasn't worth the pain to be clean of the medicine, when antidepressants can provide a floor for me to stand on and be myself.

A side effect of the antidepressants that I didn't like was the lowered libido and orgasmic ability. I went to one psychiatrist who is a specialist in hormonal women. Hormones and depression, you put them all together, and that is an issue. I now take testosterone cream that puts me back to a normal level of testosterone in my body. But my major discovery has been gingko biloba. Taking 240 mg of gingko biloba a day has provided an antidote for the negative orgasmic effects of antidepressants for me, and there are no side effects.

I've also worked with a homeopath who suggested things like chromium, and supplements that actually helped maintain my blood sugar levels. I had become a vegetarian along the way, and she challenged me not to continue doing this, saying I need more animal protein, especially with my history of depression. I avoid sugar, and eat carob now instead of chocolate; that seems to satisfy my desire for sweets.

Exercise was never a way I dealt with my eating disorder. I was almost always active, in a non-compulsive way, because I was a dancer. Then, when running got into style, I did running. I used it in the sense that I knew on the days I ran a lot, I could eat more, but I did not have that anorexic drive to push, push, push. When I was depressed, I couldn't exercise at all because I had no energy for it. These days, I exercise moderately, and it is still an issue for me about having the energy at times. I know doing aerobics would be really good for me and help me sleep better, but I do take relatively long walks four or five times a week.

I've learned to treat myself in hard times with things other than food—a massage, a nap, a long bath, a video. I depend more on myself now than I ever did. It used to be that I would have to call someone and cry to them, and now there are times that I will just hug a pillow and cry. I'm using the things that help me best, like spiritual connection, nature, close relationships, and therapy still. My job as a book editor is highly satisfying. I get to use my intellectual skills and help people at the same time. I'm always learning in this job.

I haven't stopped being self-critical completely, but I catch myself doing it a lot sooner, and the intensity and duration are both less. Occasionally I still eat emotionally, but it is almost a little joke I have with myself now. If I know I need to have some "mommy" food, or some emotional food, I eat these great treats I found that are like puffed air. It is just something I put in my mouth to soothe myself, and I know it.

Taking responsibility for my actions, but not taking blame for them, is at the very heart of recovery for me. I've become more accepting of the paradoxes in my life. Considering myself as someone who has recovered from compulsive overeating, I also know that it's an ongoing relationship between me, myself, and food. By having elimi-nated certain foods from my diet, I experience more freedom. By allowing my self-critical voices to be there at times, rather than fight them, ironically they shift faster. The forces that used to be at war with each other are finding peaceful coexistence.

8

SARA

Sara is 36 years old and married, with a 3-year-old son and a baby on the way. She works part-time in catering sales. Sara was bulimic for nine years and has been symptom-free the past six years.

I started gaining weight when I was eight years old and was pretty chubby until I turned thirteen. I know I used food for comfort at an early age. My dad was an alcoholic who often drank when he got home from work. That meant by the time our family sat down for dinner, he was in a mean mood. He never physically abused us, but he used words to pick on us and needle us. My mom has always been heavy, and he would make nasty comments about her weight. Many of our meals dissolved into tense, ugly times. My mom usually ignored him or told him to shut up, but I reacted by having second helpings.

We were actually a close family, despite a lot of dysfunction. When I was young, I didn't know my dad had a problem with alcohol; I just knew he acted funny sometimes, not quite like himself. It scared me a lot because I didn't want anything bad to happen to him. My mom worked a few nights a week and I used to worry if he was eating dinner alone that he would choke on his food and die. Many nights, my two sisters and I would literally kind of carry him off to bed, and he would usually say, "I'm dying." That would always create a sense of instability and fear for me. It ruined a lot of vacations and family times.

I think I got used to ignoring whether or not I was full because I was stuffing all my feelings down during family meals. I developed anger at my father early on, but didn't know how to express it. My mom didn't confront my father, or show much of a reaction to his behavior, so I didn't have an example to follow. My mom is one of the nicest people in the world, and she just seems to let bad behavior roll off her back. So, on the one hand, I loved my dad because in certain ways he was caring and loving, and on the other hand, I was worried and mad at him.

By the time I was in sixth grade, I was heavy enough that a boy in my class called me an elephant. I broke into tears and ran out of the room. While I cried in the bathroom, a popular girl named Melissa came in and told me she had gone up and hit this boy. That made me feel better, that someone acknowledged how cruel he was. But I definitely felt much less accepted than the girls who were thin. I was already quiet and shy around everyone but my family, and my weight made me even more self-conscious.

My sisters were both on the thin side, and could eat like horses without gaining weight. Diana is three years older than me, and Laura is two years younger. I don't remember my parents actually saying anything to me about my weight, but my dad packed our lunches most mornings, and mine was very different from my sisters'. They got two sandwiches, Ding Dongs, chips, and fruit, while all I got was half an apple and half a sandwich. In this way, he put me on a diet. But in junior high I would eat what he packed, and then go to the snack bar and get a burrito and an ice cream sandwich. So, I didn't let him stop me.

My dad enrolled us in a summer swimming program when I was eight, and in a year-round program when I was ten. We got Sundays off, and three weeks off during the summer. Once I turned thirteen, we had morning workouts before school, from 5 to 7 A.M., and then we'd go back for another workout for two and a half hours in the late afternoon. We would get home at seven-thirty at night, and then we would eat. Everything was just working out and eating, working out and eating. I really didn't like it, but I kept doing it because my dad really wanted us to swim.

There was never any time to do anything else. I was a good swimmer, but I knew I was never going to be really good like my older sister.

Finally, it just became too serious and competitive, and I wasn't getting much out of it. I hated when my dad would come into the room at 4:30 A.M. to get us up for practice. I would just cringe.

I got the nerve up to quit when I was fifteen. My coach made me feel like I was really bad for quitting, and so did my dad. I felt somewhat lost and bad about myself for a while. I hadn't made any friends at school. My swimming friends were a tight-knit group, and my first dance, my first kiss, my first everything, was with the swim team kids. It took me until my junior year in high school to make my first school friend.

Because I was so quiet and shy in high school, I thought taking drama class would force me out of my shell. When I was younger, before swimming consumed my life, I used to get together with friends and write, direct, and perform plays. But when I told my dad I wanted to do drama instead of swimming, he told me that was a dumb idea. I never tried it because he said that. I hate the fact that I let his words affect me so much, that I did not even try something.

My older sister, Diana, excelled in everything she did—school, swimming, making friends, and being thin. I don't think I was actually jealous of her, because we were so close and I was proud of her. But I know I compared myself to her all the time, and felt like I didn't measure up. My self-esteem wasn't very high. I was still a bit heavy, about fifteen pounds more than I wanted to be.

When I graduated from high school, I enrolled in a junior college, and became friends with a girl who did drugs. Before then, I drank in my senior year a bit, but I hadn't done any drugs. She turned me on to crank. It made me talk more and be more outgoing, which is what I'd always wanted to do. Soon it became my escape, and I would be up all night three or four nights a week. I lost a bunch of weight, but I started getting really irritable. After a year of doing crank, I didn't like it much anymore, but I just couldn't stop. One night, I got into a huge fight with my dad, and I started having a fit. He had to literally pick me up and hold me down just to try to calm me. When I finally quit, I slept about twenty hours straight and spent three days trying to detox. It was such a high just to be normal again.

I went back to eating, though, and ballooned up to 168 pounds. I'm 5'6" so it wasn't huge, but it was heavier than a lot of people. I was twenty-one at the time, and a girlfriend had asked me to be the maid of honor in her wedding. I thought, "I'm not going to be in a wedding looking like this," so I went to Jenny Craig, and I started running a lot. I ran about four miles a day, but if I went off my diet and ate a brownie, I'd run an extra three miles to burn it off. Jenny Craig diets were about 1,000 calories, or maybe 1,200. It was nothing. I lost about twenty-five pounds in four months.

Then, about a month before the wedding, my parents had a big Easter feast. They had a huge spread of food that I loved, and I just kept eating all day long. I felt panicked at the end of the afternoon and remembered reading in a magazine a technique to make yourself throw up. It wasn't sticking your finger down your throat; it was drinking soda. So I drank some soda, went and leaned over the toilet, and pushed on my stomach. The food just came up, and I was so relieved. I didn't feel panic any more.

I started this once a day, or every other day if I felt myself get full. But I knew it wasn't healthy and that I should tell someone. So I told my mom, and I don't think she knew what to say. She just said, "Well, don't do that anymore. It's bad for you." I think she asked me about it one time after that, and I just lied. It never got brought up again, and I just got worse and worse.

I think being bulimic had a lot to do with how I looked. I had lost weight, and suddenly got all this attention from guys because I looked better. I had always identified being liked and accepted with being thin. Now that I felt better about my appearance, I worried that I would balloon up again. So I kept being bulimic. I didn't really lose weight this way, but I was able to maintain it.

About six months after I started the bulimia, I got involved with a married man. I just started making decisions in my life that kind of fed the low self-esteem issue. It was my first love, my first relationship. I met him at a concert and didn't know he was married at first. He was with some other guys and wasn't wearing a wedding band. We got to talking and just clicked. But I soon found out he was married and had a little boy. He was devoted to his son and didn't want to break up his marriage, but he said he didn't love his wife anymore.

I had started a job managing a small restaurant that served breakfast and lunch, and had moved into my own apartment before I met John. He was a graphic artist. We used to get together at my apartment a few nights a week and whenever we could on weekends. Sometimes, we went away together on weekends. I genuinely loved him, and I know he really loved me too. To this day, I know it. It felt like my heart came home when I was sitting next to him. But I also knew this was all wrong, and that even if he left his wife, it would never be right. So, while there were wonderful, loving moments in our relationship, there were also icky, negative ones. I resented the time he spent with his wife, but I also felt guilty all the time about being involved with him.

All these mixed emotions just kept feeding the bulimia. I started every day thinking, "I am not going to do it." I would go to work and not eat very much. I was pretty hungry by the time I was through with work, at about 2:30 P.M., and I would bring a healthy lunch home from the restaurant. But when I ate it, I'd feel too full, and then have panicky feelings about gaining all the weight back again. So I would get rid of it, and feel bad about myself, and that would trigger going to the store to get more food.

I went to different grocery stores since I was afraid people would recognize that I was just there the day before. I bought anything I wanted—donuts, ice cream, pancake mix, cookies, chips, cereal, and also some healthy food like eggs and salad stuff. Sometimes I binged and purged for five to six hours at a time. One binge triggered another. Even though I ate some healthy food mixed in with the junk, I'd throw that up too. I didn't have any outside interests except my job and John. Since he usually couldn't spend much time with me, I had lots of time on my hands. I was disgusted with myself, and was spending all my money on food that I wasn't even keeping down. And I couldn't tell anyone about my bulimia; it was too shameful.

I knew I couldn't go on like this, and I finally decided to get some help. My first attempt to actually tell someone was awful. I was in my own little apartment, all alone, and I called a doctor on my health plan. I said I needed some help, and I remember having a hard time saying the word "bulimia" over the phone. He said, "What is that?" and I said, "I eat and throw up." My face was turning red, I was so embarrassed to say it. He told me he couldn't fit me in for two months. I asked if he had any advice about what I could do in the meantime, and he suggested the Atkins diet.

I knew that wasn't going to work, so I tried someone else. I heard a therapist speak on a local talk show, and went to see him for counseling. He was really down on my relationship with John, and I felt really judged. I did not need someone telling me what was wrong with the relationship; it wasn't the way to help me. Finally, I confided in a younger coworker who was anorexic, and she recommended the therapist she was seeing. This one specialized in treating eating disorders, and I immediately felt more comfortable and accepted.

Gradually, I learned more about myself, and how to recognize and deal with my feelings. I used to think I was a lazy person and get on myself about all that I did wrong. In therapy I learned how to be easier on myself in certain ways, and kinder to myself. My self-esteem improved. Of course, no one knew that I didn't look as good on the inside as I did on the outside. When I was able to reduce the bingeing and purging, I started feeling better about myself. It goes hand in hand; you binge and purge because of low self-esteem, but it goes even lower when you do it. It was like a snowball effect. I exercised by running a few miles a day as often as I could. I tried not to criticize myself for being lazy on the days when I just didn't feel like exercising.

Finally, after over four years of being together, I broke up with John. We had gone away for a weekend, and his wife kept calling him at the hotel. He said he had to take the calls, and I had no tolerance for it, none. I was tired of waiting for him to leave his wife, and I didn't believe it would ever happen. It was hard at first, but I quickly met other guys who were interested in me. And I spent more time with my family and girlfriends. I made better choices in people and relationships, and also in how I spent my time.

My next relationship was a much healthier one. By then, I knew that I had a pattern of getting involved with men who were not fully emotionally available, going back to my dad and his alcoholism. When I met Nick, my first instinct was it wasn't a match. But he was such a nice person, and treated me so wonderfully, that I made a conscious decision to break my pattern. I made myself look into this relationship, even though it was very uncomfortable at first. I was used to having chemistry lead the way, and that wasn't the case with Nick. I began to love him very much, but it never seemed like that lifelong kind of love. We were close, though, and I was able to tell him about my eating disorder. It was a good step for me to be able to level with someone. I basically told him that I didn't want to keep it from him, but that it was something I had to deal with, and I didn't want him asking me about it

We lived together for two years, but he got on my nerves really easily. I didn't want to spend my life like that, being dissatisfied with so many minor things. My bulimia started tapering off, and I got into a strict eating and exercise program. I began working with a trainer and got into really good shape. If I overate a little bit, I would still get rid of it, but I didn't have huge binges anymore. Eventually I ended it with Nick, but even now, years later, we're still on friendly terms.

Indirectly, Nick had a big part in my recovery from bulimia. His part-time housekeeper was a very religious Christian lady. One day a few months after Nick and I broke up, she showed up at the restaurant where I worked, and said she had been thinking of me. I didn't know her that well, so it was a bit odd. She invited me to join her Bible study group, and I decided to give it a try. I had already been reading some spiritual books, trying to find some peace and guidance. In this church group, we took a section of the Bible each week, and went home and thought about how it related to our lives. Then we'd come back and discuss it with each other. After that, there was a lecture for the last forty-five minutes or so.

Well, one day after I'd been attending the Bible study classes for almost a year, the lecture at the end had to do with finding comfort in God and Jesus. The last question of the evening was, "Who do you turn to for counsel or comfort?" I looked up in church and thought, "Oh my God. I have been trying to fix myself, and I have been going to every person with knowledge and books so that someone can fix me. But I never just turned to you." I had a sense of peace come over me in that pew, and I went home, and I have never thrown up since.

I had figured out a lot of stuff in the counseling, but I was still purging at times. All I know is that at that moment in church, I surrendered the last traces of this habit and it was just gone. I think I had a void to fill, with something other than food. Every day kind of went by, and I chose not to do it any more. When I felt full and got that panicky feeling, I sat with myself, and I sat with the feelings that went along with the anxiety and panic. I knew I was not going to gain twenty pounds because I ate a burrito or a piece of candy. My life was not going to end. It gave me a lot of confidence to sit with myself and let these uncomfortable feelings pass. I kept thinking, "They passed this time and they will pass the next time." I knew as long as I ate reasonably, I was not going to put on weight. I finally became proud of myself.

It felt like a reward when I met my husband soon after I stopped being bulimic. We met through one of my cousins, and he was all the good things in my past relationships wrapped up into one person. I felt comfortable with him immediately. He is loyal and stable and loving, and I know we belong together.

Our little boy is the light of our lives, and we're excited about our baby that's due in a few months. I do still have those patterns that I used to have, when I'm feeling stressed and can easily turn to food. It's a conscious thing now. I have to say to myself, "Okay, I really feel like having the chicken sandwich with the cheese and onions and butter, but I am going to have the salad with the tuna because I don't want to get huge with this pregnancy." I know I'm the type of person who can gain weight easily, so I need to watch what I eat and exercise. I find that when I don't exercise, my eating patterns get worse, so I make sure I go to the gym or run or walk almost every day.

My confidence level is still definitely affected by my weight. But at least I know that if I were ever to lapse back into the bulimia, I would be able to get out of it again. Before, I didn't have that level of confidence, but now I do. I still struggle, like a lot of people do, with trying to be happy. We have financial worries, some extended family issues, and the usual day-to-day problems. I think we grow up thinking there's an end to the rainbow, when there's really not. I thought I'd get to a point where I'd always be happy, but of course that isn't possible. There is always a new challenge, but I know I can depend on myself, my spiritual beliefs, and people who love me to help with the rough times.

9

WHAT TO DO IF YOU HAVE AN EATING DISORDER

The personal stories in the preceding chapters illustrate just how difficult it can be to finally attain physical and emotional health. Though each person chose a unique path, there are some essential steps to consider if you are suffering from an eating disorder. But first we will explore why it is difficult to seek any treatment at all—or even tell anyone you have this problem—and how to motivate yourself to take action.

Although you know you are having difficulties with food and body image, you will probably deny you have a problem if asked. You are most likely a private person who wants to be independent and in control. You fear embarrassment and intrusion into your personal life. If you are like the majority of people I have treated, you believe you can figure out your own solutions to the problem and you want to be left alone. You may be a strong-willed person in many other areas and are now full of frustration and self-loathing that you are eating out of control. Or you may be happily anorexic, feeling proud and strong that you can resist food and be thinner than others.

You have developed the symptoms of an eating disorder for a reason. It serves a purpose for you. As previously mentioned, many people start off wanting to lose weight to feel better about themselves and their bodies. You may find you enjoy the admiration and attention you receive from others, as well as increased self-regard. You may ultimately become hooked on the feelings of control and mastery associated with dieting. If you continue restricting your food intake, you feel stronger and stronger. If you are unable to continue restricting, you feel like a failure, and you may binge or overeat out of a need for temporary comfort and distraction.

Perhaps bingeing, purging, and obsessing about food helps numb you to emotional pain you carry deep inside. Some patients I have treated were sexually molested by a family member, neighbor, or friend. There seem to be increasing numbers of women who are victims of date rape. Sometimes there is pain over the loss of a parent or a divorce. There can be pain resulting from parental neglect or emotional or physical abuse by a parent or loved ones.

One woman I worked with for three years, whom I'll call Claire, suffered from compulsive overeating and bouts of bulimia. Initially, she viewed her problems with food as the result of dissatisfaction with being overweight most of her life. After some time in therapy, Claire began to realize that her parents' emphasis on appearances—hers, theirs, and others'—caused her great anger, distress, and hurt. Because she loved her parents and wanted to have a close relationship with them, Claire buried these negative feelings and stuffed herself with food just as she stuffed down her feelings. Eventually, she came to terms with her ambivalence toward her parents and their values, and she mourned the loss of her idealized notion that she had accepting, nurturing parents. She worked on maintaining a good relationship with them, nonetheless, since that was her desire. Gradually, Claire was able to develop more self-discipline with food and exercise as she gained greater clarity in her life.

Another patient, "Meredith," had repressed several instances of molestation by an uncle when she was seven and eight years old. She entered therapy to gain control over her long-term problem with bulimia and to learn tips on how to handle certain trigger foods. As difficult as it was for Meredith to uncover what propelled her eating disorder, in the process she was able to experience vindication and release from the quagmire of self-destructive thoughts and behavior.

Steps to Overcome Your Eating Disorder:

Awareness

If you have an eating disorder and are reading this book, this is a good sign. It means that you are curious about what others have experienced and that you realize something is not quite right with your own life. The first step is always *awareness*. Once you become aware of a problem, you can begin to gather information for yourself. You can read books and articles, use the Web for information and chat rooms, watch TV specials and talk shows that address the subject, and tune into others around you who mention having problems with food.

Tell Someone

The stage of gathering information may last for quite some time before you are ready to admit to yourself and others that you need help. Many of my patients have talked about how scary it is at first to tell their doctor or confide in a therapist who is a stranger at first. Often, they had not told anyone else—parents, spouse, or friends—about their eating disorder. This step is the hardest for many people. It is important that you stop harboring this secret. Maintaining a façade that everything is fine can be extremely difficult and depleting. You need support and reassurance so that you can feel acceptance despite having a problem. The mere act of telling someone is often liberating and can help set you on the path to recovery.

Seek Help

The next step is crucial. This is when you shift from thinking that the problem will eventually go away, or that you can handle it alone, to going to a professional for help. Invariably, people who are hesitant to seek help become motivated to do so when they experience serious problems related to their eating disorder. A common term for this stage is "hitting bottom." Some have lost their jobs because of absenteeism or erratic performance; some have jeopardized relationships; some have experienced worrisome health or dental problems; and some are simply exhausted from the ups and downs of an eating disorder.

Very few people are able to recover from an eating disorder without some sort of professional help. Laura, in Chapter Two, did not get help because of financial concerns, but after enduring her problems for so many years, she gives advice to others to get professional help or join a group. Why prolong the unhappiness, when it gets to that point, and deny yourself some support? The fact is that the longer you allow your eating disorder to go untreated, the longer the recovery process will be.

Some people begin to get help by seeing their physician for a checkup and then confiding their problem. Most physicians are knowledgeable about eating disorders and can provide a referral to a therapist. It is important to work with a therapist who specializes in treating eating disorders. There are many capable therapists to choose from, but only those who specialize in this area can offer the comprehensive treatment you need.

Selecting a Therapist

You can obtain names of therapists specializing in the area of eating disorders from your physician, your local hospitals, personal contacts, and referral Web sites (see Resource List). If you are a student or can only afford low-fee therapy, college counseling centers often offer assistance; however, you will need to ask specifically for someone who is knowledgeable about eating disorders.

It is a good idea to interview the therapist before you commit to treatment. You are the "shopper," and it is important that you not only feel comfortable talking to this individual, but that you also have confidence he or she can help you. Some questions you might ask include the following:

- How long will therapy last, and how many sessions per week are recommended?

- What are the therapist's credentials, licenses, and experiences in treating eating disorders?

- What are the fees, and what are the terms for contact between sessions if necessary?

- Exactly how does the therapist plan to help you?

- What approach does the therapist use? Some possibilities include the following:

  - Psychodynamic: Focuses on uncovering unconscious motives and influences to eliminate self-deception and conflict. Usually long-term.

  - Jungian: Fosters awareness of how our inner and outer worlds relate. Promotes an inner journey of self-discovery and personal meaning. Usually long-term.

  - Cognitive: Helps patients modify thoughts and behavior by examining self-defeating thinking.

  - Behavioral: Targets observable and measurable behaviors to modify.

  - Eclectic: Combines two or more therapeutic approaches. Many therapists employ a variety of methods in treating patients.

Most eating disorder therapists use a team approach to helping a patient. They work closely with physicians, psychiatrists, and nutritionists, as well as family therapists when that work is indicated. They will help coordinate your treatment so that all of the necessary concerns are addressed. If you haven't already consulted a physician, your therapist will recommend that you do so. If you are suffering from signs of severe depression and are receptive to the possibility of trying an antidepressant, your therapist will recommend a consultation with a psychiatrist. If you are strongly opposed to taking medication, your therapist will respect your decision, even though she may try to persuade you to at least give it a trial period during the course of your treatment.

An essential component of any eating disorder treatment team is the nutritionist. You will need to work with a nutritionist who specializes in treating eating disorders. Most nutritionists are highly knowledgeable about the body and its nutritional requirements, but those who specialize in eating disorders can help more effectively with the food phobias, insecurities, fears, and myths that surround this disorder. Working weekly with a nutritionist provides another layer of support, reassurance, and feedback in your efforts to become healthy.

Medication

Generally speaking, antidepressant medication helps people avoid the kind of deep despair that interferes with their ability to function properly. Antidepressants can improve sleep, increase energy levels and concentration, and help avoid feelings of overwhelming negativity.

There are several misconceptions about antidepressants. They are not "happy pills" that automatically produce a feeling of well-being. They do not insulate you from feeling pain or loss, or from experiencing appropriate reactions to life events, and they are not addictive. If you are diagnosed with depression, a psychiatrist will recommend medication for a period of time, with periodic check-ins for dosage adjustment and monitoring. You and your psychiatrist will then work together to determine how long you will remain on medication.

Whether or not to take medication is a highly personal decision. If you have underlying depression as well as an eating disorder, you will make faster progress in your recovery if you address all of your symptoms. Fortunately, there are increasing numbers of antidepressant medications that are effective and have no significant side effects.

Group or Individual Therapy?

If you are just beginning to seek treatment, you may think group therapy is the best option. It is more cost-effective and offers more opportunities for support than working with just one therapist. For many years I ran eating disorders groups composed of some members who were in individual therapy and some who were not. I noticed that the patients who made the most progress were those who combined both group *and* individual therapy.

Groups are an effective form of treatment, either in conjunction with individual therapy or as a follow-up, maintenance approach to your therapy. But I do not recommend them as a substitute for personal therapy. Through the intimate and trusting relationship you establish with your individual therapist, you gain access to a safe environment for exploring your underlying feelings and thoughts. Trying to relate to four to six other people in a group and share therapy time with them can delay your exploration or even inhibit it. I suggest waiting to join a group until you have some basic insights into yourself and the motivations behind your eating disorder.

Exercise

You have read in some of the preceding chapters how several people became compulsive exercisers. Learning how to exercise moderately and healthfully is important in your recovery. We know that regular exercise increases our production of endorphins, brain chemicals that create feelings of well-being. Exercising consistently gives us a sense of accomplishment because we are doing something positive for ourselves. It helps regulate our eating and sleeping, and improves our body image and overall health.

One of my patients, Amanda, took an "all-or-nothing" approach to exercise. She set a goal for herself of going to the gym six times a week. If she missed a few days, leaving only three possible days to exercise, for example, she got discouraged and frustrated with herself and didn't go to the gym at all. Having rigid expectations interfered with Amanda's ability to incorporate regular exercise into her life. In the course of our work together, she was able to accept that going to the gym even a few days a week was still quite helpful. She learned to feel proud of herself when she did something positive, such as exercising, and how to resist self-critical thoughts.

If you are anorexic, it is essential that you stop all exercise until your physician determines your health is no longer in jeopardy. When you are cleared for exercise, you will need to start slowly and increase the level very gradually so as not to put too much stress on your heart and other organs. Because overexercising is part of the disease process, you may have a difficult time trying to stop or reduce it on your own. You will probably need intervention and a great deal of support.

Support

This part is often difficult for many people. Revealing your emotions to others means risking possible embarrassment or rejection. Choosing to keep most of your pain and unhappiness private may feel more comfortable. It is difficult to determine the true extent of eating disorders in our society because so many people keep their problem hidden.

The recovery process invariably involves confiding in others. To begin, you will need to disclose your thoughts, feelings, and history to your team of professionals to make progress in your treatment. For many, this is much easier than telling family or friends, but it is important to eventually acknowledge your problem to some of the people with whom you have close ties. It is a healthy step to let some people in your life know "the real you." You will be able to be yourself and drop pretenses, excuses, and lies. You will be able to let go of much of your guilt about deceiving and disappointing others.

In addition to therapy groups, community-based groups provide additional support. Overeaters Anonymous offers free support groups in most communities. The groups operate on the model of Alcoholics Anonymous in which members receive a sponsor who is far enough along in her own recovery to help others effectively. In addition, online eating disorder support groups and chat rooms can be valuable resources, and they are available at all times.

To take advantage of these tools for recovery, you will need to remind yourself that you not only need help, but that you *deserve* help. There is nothing weak about needing and accepting help; as a matter of fact, it is a *strength* to be able to do this. Most of my patients start out with a double standard for themselves and others. They tell me that if they were advising a friend or relative, they would insist that she get help and take care of herself. But as for themselves—they should be able to handle this on their own. The higher standard they impose on themselves interferes with their own intuition and common sense. In urging you to seek help, I ask you to consider a variation of the Golden Rule: "Do unto yourself as you would have others do unto themselves." It is my hope that you will not delay in taking the necessary steps to help yourself both physically and emotionally.

10

WHAT TO DO IF SOMEONE YOU LOVE HAS AN EATING DISORDER

If you are a relative or friend of someone with an eating disorder, you may be uncertain about how you can help. Friends and siblings sometimes promise to keep this problem a secret and then feel prohibited from sharing the burden or seeking help from others. This is always a mistake. It is imperative that you tell people who can help your loved one. It is better to risk her anger than to silently stand by while she jeopardizes her health. It is also not fair to burden yourself with such a huge responsibility. As they progress in their treatment, patients tell me that they are very grateful and relieved that their friend or sibling told someone who could get them help.

Each person reacts in his or her own way to the alarming problem of a loved one with an eating disorder. The mother of one anorexic patient emotionally withdrew, both from her daughter and from the entire family during the first year of her daughter's treatment. She later described in family work how difficult it was to fake being strong and confident when inside she felt like she was falling apart. She felt too guilty and awful about herself and her failings as a mother to talk to anyone about these feelings. This mother's withdrawal created not just a burden for her, but also for my patient, who then felt intensified guilt and responsibility for causing such pain to her family.

Sometimes parents react to their child's problem by blaming each other, as well as their child. The ways of expressing this anger vary.

Some are able to talk about it; others suppress their feelings and may act out in passive-aggressive ways toward their spouse and child. One father kept forgetting to pick up his daughter from therapy appointments or to be home on time for family social occasions. Later, he was able to look at his behavior and realize how angry he was at his wife. He felt his wife had always spoiled their daughter, and now their daughter had severe bulimia. He blamed them both for causing him such unhappiness and worry.

Another family reacted in an extreme way to their daughter's bulimia. Daria binged constantly, eating everything in the refrigerator and pantry. She even ate cans of vegetables and fruits. The family was furious with her when she ate the leftovers they planned to have for another meal and when she ate some of the ingredients they counted on using for that night's dinner. As a result, Daria's parents put a padlock on the refrigerator and the pantry door. While this method protected their food, it only served to enrage Daria. She felt demeaned and shamed. She couldn't have friends over because it would have been too difficult to try to explain the locks. She resorted to stealing money from her parents to spend on food, and even stealing food from stores.

These examples of family struggles highlight the need for family therapy and support groups while a beloved child is in the throes of an eating disorder. Here are a few basic guidelines to help you through this difficult time: (For purposes of simplification, I will refer to the individual with the eating disorder as your daughter, although your loved one may be male and a sibling, spouse, other relative, or friend.)

- *First, it is important to realize that there are no quick or easy solutions to an eating disorder.* Most eating disorders, even with treatment, persist for months and even years. It takes time to find the best help and methods to assist in your loved one's recovery. You need to educate yourself about the various options, and help pave the way for her to enter treatment.

- *If your child is younger than eighteen, insist that she have a medical and psychological assessment by practitioners experienced in eating disorders.* Be loving, but forceful, in making sure she participates in ongoing therapy. If she is over eighteen, you need to exert whatever power you have to make sure she gets help. Some families have refused to continue paying for college unless their child sees a therapist and has regular medical exams. They also insist that their child give authorization for them to have contact with the professionals involved in her treatment.

- *Learn to take care of yourself.* Do not let your life or your family members' lives revolve around the eating disorder or the sick person. You will end up feeling exhausted and resentful. Of course, there will be a certain amount of worry and frustration, but try to include satisfying activities and fun in your life. Some families feel like withdrawing from the world, but this is a time when it is especially important to maintain outside relationships and interests. To do so sets a good example for your daughter. She will benefit from your strength during this difficult time.

- *Don't dwell on feelings of guilt or self-blame.* Recognize that your daughter's behavior is likely to cause you to feel helpless, fearful, frustrated, and possibly angry as well. Don't expect yourself to be completely loving and accepting at all times. That is a setup for failure. Most parents want to know what they have done wrong and how they may have contributed to the development of their child's eating disorder. Remember that eating disorders stem from different combinations of factors—possibly biological, psychological, social, and/or familial. There are no perfect parents or perfect families. Understanding family dynamics is important, but dwelling on guilt or blame can be depleting and counterproductive.

- *Find a support group or your own counseling to help you cope. Family therapy is also important; having a child with any disease or disorder puts stress on a marriage, as well as on the entire family.* Family therapy not only helps the patient, but the entire family, who benefit from greater communication and understanding. Families also need to learn about eating disorders by reading relevant literature and consulting with professionals. The resource list in the back of this book offers contact information for eating disorder organizations, as well as some helpful book suggestions.

- *Avoid letting your child's peculiar eating habits and food choices dominate your household, but be responsive to her needs.* Your child should not dictate what your family eats, which restaurants you patronize, or where you go on vacations. At the same time, because she is a member of the family, it is important to consider her preferences and needs along with everyone else's. Families are usually cooperative in removing tempting binge foods from easy access. It is a similar concept to removing alcohol when a family member is in the process of recovering from alcoholism. Families can limit tempting foods in the kitchen and the rest of the house, and may even put their own snack foods in a locked cabinet in the garage or bedroom. The most common binge foods are sweets and carbohydrates. You can't prevent your child from mixing up a batch of pancakes, but you can help her by not having sweets readily available. I recommend that parents and siblings go out for ice cream or a dessert when they want and be sure to make available a variety of foods that feel safe to your loved one.

- *Let your daughter know how much you love and appreciate her.* Let her hear how you value her for all of her intrinsic qualities, rather than just for her accomplishments, performance, or appearance. For example, when you see demonstrations of her good sense of humor or compassion for others, let her know you think these traits are special. Don't compare her to anyone else. She needs to feel a greater sense of herself and her own worth.

- *Minimize comments, discussions, or arguments with her about food, weight, and her appearance.* Even if your anorexic daughter has finally gained some weight, do not tell her she looks better or healthy. She will usually interpret this remark to mean she is now fat. Your daughter will invariably have a great deal of anxiety about her eating and her appearance. You can offer reassurance, but it is often best for the nutritionist and therapist to serve as sounding boards for these fears and anxieties. This preserves your energy to deal with all of the other issues that go along with parenting a child.

- *Hold your daughter accountable for her behavior.* Do not be afraid of setting limits and upsetting her, thinking your actions will cause her to become more entrenched in her eating disorder. She is feeling out-of-control in general, so it will help her to have structure with consistent limits and consequences. You cannot allow yourself, as a parent, to be held hostage by her eating disorder.

- *If you become concerned about weight loss, dehydration, or other medical problems, call her physician or therapist.* If she refuses treatment and her health is in jeopardy, you will need to obtain help in physically transporting her to a hospital. Some parents must do this several times during the course of their child's eating disorder.

- *Realize that your child may be ambivalent about wanting to get well.* Sometimes she may try hard to be healthy; at other times, she will retreat into the relative safety and comfort of her rituals or bizarre food behaviors. Ambivalence and inconsistency are inherent in the struggle to overcome an eating disorder.

- *Recognize that relapsing is part of the recovery process.* Try not to become discouraged or to convey discouragement to your daughter. Any behavioral change consists of some steps up, some steps down, and some plateaus. Continue to get support for yourself so that you can better tolerate the inevitable fluctuations in your child's path to recovery.

CONCLUSION

You have read how seven individuals struggled and triumphed over their eating disorders. Now think about which story or part of a story sparked a light of identification and understanding for you. What feelings did you come away with after you finished reading these stories? It may be helpful to go back and reread the stories that affected you the most. In addition, talking to someone about your reactions or writing down your thoughts and feelings on paper or in a journal can be therapeutic tools for your own recovery process.

Although each story is unique, there are many common threads. Not only did all seven people experience distress and fear over food and weight gain, but they also developed a secondary set of negative feelings about themselves. With so many complex factors involved, it is understandable why recovering from an eating disorder is not just a simple process. Here are some emotional side effects that usually develop in a pronounced way:

- *Self-loathing.* Some of the people relating their stories initially had shaky self-esteem and personal dissatisfactions, but they did not feel such intense anger and revulsion toward themselves until the onset of the eating disorder. Then, if they ate more than they planned, they were "pigs" and "disgusting." If they didn't exercise as intended, or if they procrastinated at times, they were "lazy." If they avoided social contact, they were "bad." If they couldn't concentrate in school, they were "stupid." People with eating disorders would not condemn friends or others in this harsh way, yet sadly they do it to themselves.

- *Guilt.* Not only did they feel guilty when they ate certain foods or ate more food than they intended, but then another layer of guilt set in. There was guilt over causing loved ones worry, unhappiness, and financial strain. There was guilt over being too needy or too dependent. There was guilt over being too avoidant and antisocial. Guilt can spread like a virus and permeate every facet of our lives. A certain amount of guilt can help guide us, but too much can become overwhelming and demoralizing.

- *Worry and anxiety*. A worry or fear has a specific focus, whereas anxiety is vague and undefined. It is easy to see how worry and anxiety set in when people feel trapped by their eating disorders. Some of the worries expressed in these stories, besides the looming ones related to food and weight, concerned issues of health, fertility, self-sufficiency, finances, intimacy, and loneliness. An overlay of worry and anxiety can complicate recovery from an eating disorder.

If you are experiencing some of these negative emotions, as well as an eating disorder, it is time for you to take action. You need to eliminate "magical thinking"—that as soon as you get a new job, find a boyfriend, lose twenty pounds, and save some money, *then* your life will be fine. You need to consider how much of your life you are wasting, feeling stuck or depressed and hopeless, unable to make progress and achieve growth. You need to consider how many people *do* care about you and all that you *do* have going for you, instead of looking at the proverbial cup as half empty.

Each individual in this book endured years of disordered eating and unhappiness. The longer an eating disorder goes untreated, the longer the period of recovery can be. If you see early signs of an eating disorder in yourself or in a loved one, don't delay in consulting your physician or a therapist. If you are already struggling with anorexia, bulimia, or compulsive overeating, remember that if you make a determined effort, you *will* become healthy. Healing can start with just one small step at a time. If you persevere, as these seven people did, and do not let yourself become discouraged by the up-and-down nature of recovery, you too will ultimately achieve self-acceptance and contentment.

APPENDIX

Sources and Suggested Reading:

Bruch, Hilde. *The Golden Cage: The Enigma of Anorexia Nervosa*. Harvard University Press, 1978.

Bryant-Waugh, Rachel, and Bryan Lask. *Eating Disorders: A Parent's Guide*. Brunner-Routledge, 2004.

Chernin, Kim. *The Obsession: Reflections on the Tyranny of Slenderness*. Harper & Row, 1981.

Collins, Laura. *Eating with Your Anorexic: How My Child Recovered through Family-Based Treatment and Yours Can Too*. McGraw-Hill, 2005.

Costin, Carolyn. *The Eating Disorder Sourcebook: A Comprehensive Guide to the Causes, Treatments, and Prevention of Eating Disorders*. Lowell House, 1999.

Fallon, Patricia, Melanie Katzman, and Susan Wooley. *Feminist Perspectives on Eating Disorders*. The Guilford Press, 1994.

Garner, David, and Paul Garfinkel. *Handbook of Treatment for Eating Disorders*. Guilford Press, 1997.

Hall, Lindsey, and Leigh Cohn. *Bulimia: A Guide to Recovery*. Gurze Books, 1999.

———. *Anorexia Nervosa: A Guide to Recovery*. Gurze Books, 1999.

Hirschmann, Jane R., and Carol Munter. *When Women Stop Hating Their Bodies: Freeing Yourself from Food and Weight Obsession.* Fawcett Columbine, 1995.

Hornbacher, Marya. *Wasted: A Memoir of Anorexia and Bulimia.* Harper Perennial, 1998.

Ikeda, Joanne P. *Am I Fat? Helping Children Accept Differences in Body Size.* ETR Associates, 1992.

Katherine, Anne. *Anatomy of a Food Addiction.* Gurze Books, 1991.

Lock, James, and Daniel LeGrange. *Help Your Teenager Beat an Eating Disorder.* Guilford Press, 2004.

Maine, Margo. *Body Wars: Making Peace with Women's Bodies.* Gurze Books, 1999.

Minuchin, Salvador, Bernice L. Rosman, and Lester Baker. *Psychosomatic Families: Anorexia Nervosa in Context.* Harvard University Press, 1978.

Nash, Joyce D. *Binge No More: Your Guide to Overcoming Disordered Eating.* New Harbinger Publications, 1999.

Normandi, Carol Emery, and Laurelee Roark. *It's Not about Food: End Your Obsession with Food and Weight.* Penguin Putnam, 1996.

Paulson, Tony, and Johanna Marie McShane. *Because I Feel Fat: Helping the Ones You Love Deal with an Eating Disorder.* iUniverse, 2004.

Pipher, Mary. *Hunger Pains: The Modern Woman's Tragic Quest for Thinness.* Ballantine Books, 1995.

Rodin, Judith. *Body Traps: Breaking the Binds that Keep You from Feeling Good about Your Body.* Morrow, 1992.

Roth, Geneen. *Feeding the Hungry Heart: The Experience of Compulsive Eating.* Signet, 1983.

———. *Breaking Free from Compulsive Eating.* Signet, 1986.

———. *Why Weight? A Guide to Ending Compulsive Eating.* Penguin Books, 1989.

———. *When Food Is Love: Exploring the Relationship between Eating and Intimacy.* Penguin Books, 1991.

Schaefer, Jenni, and Thom Rutledge. *Life without Ed: How One Woman Declared Independence from her Eating Disorder and You Can Too.* McGraw-Hill, 2003.

Waterhouse, Debra. *Like Mother, Like Daughter: How Women Are Influenced by Their Mother's Relationship with Food and How to Break the Pattern.* Hyperion, 1997.

Woodman, Marion. *Addiction to Perfection: The Still Unravished Bride.* Inner City Books, 1982.

———. *The Owl Was a Baker's Daughter: Obesity, Anorexia Nervosa and the Repressed Feminine.* Inner City Books, 1980.

Online Resources:

The Academy for Eating Disorders (www.aedweb.org). International transdisciplinary professional organization.

The Alliance for Eating Disorder Awareness (www. eatingdisorderinfo.org). Information, news, and treatment referral.

Anorexia Nervosa and Related Eating Disorders (ANRED) (www.anred.com). Eating disorders education and recovery information.

Eating Disorders Coalition (www.eatingdisorderscoalition.org). Works to advance recognition of eating disorders as a public health priority.

Eating Disorder Referral and Information Center (www. edreferral.org). Information and treatment referral.

Gurze Eating Disorder Resources (www.gurze.com). Lists available books and publications on eating disorders, body image, and related subjects.

National Association of Anorexia Nervosa and Associated Disorders (ANAD) (www.anad.org). Nonprofit organization offering referrals information and consumer advocacy.

National Eating Disorders Association (www. nationaleatingdisorders.org). National nonprofit organization providing information, treatment referrals, and research grants.

Overeaters Anonymous (www.oa.com). A 12-step, self-help organization based on the concepts of Alcoholics Anonymous.

About the Author

Margie Ryerson, MS, MFT, is a California marriage and family therapist who specializes in the treatment of eating disorders. She has written for professional journals and newspapers, and has lectured widely in her field.

978-0-595-34755-1
0-595-34755-X

Printed in the United Kingdom
by Lightning Source UK Ltd.
124901UK00001B/333/A